I will not give up on my Daughter

A true account of a family living with Anorexia Nervosa.

All names have been changed for privacy.
All events are true and based around a 13 year old girl named Summer who develops Anorexia Nervosa.
All members of the family have contributed to the writings.
Weights have been omitted for the benefit of Summer and for those who may find the facts triggering.

I will not give up on my daughter:
A true account of a family living with Anorexia Nervosa.

This edition published 2013

1. Mental health 2. Anorexia Nervosa 3. Patients 4. Auto Biography 5.Family
6. Self Help

Disclaimer
While every care has been taken in researching and compiling the information in this book, it is in no way intended to replace professional medical, legal advice and counselling. Readers are encouraged to seek such help as they deem necessary. The authors and publisher specifically disclaim any liability arising from the application of information in this book.

ISBN 978-0-9923531-0-0 (paperback)

All drawings, photographs and poems were submitted by the family.
There are no pictures of the family involved.

Printed and bound in Australia by Digital Creative Services.

I Wish to Acknowledge

I thank all of you who prayed for Summer and my family. I thank those who made us dinners in readiness for when we came home late from the hospital on Monday evenings. I thank my family for phoning me just to say hello and to see how things were going. I thank my friends who sent thinking of you cards and flowers. I thank my children Mia and James for accepting this challenging time and trusting that Derek and I were taking care of Summer. I also thank my gorgeous two children for continuing to love Summer even when she was at her most aggressive and destructive stage.

I thank my husband Derek for giving me hugs when I clearly looked like I needed them and although he was as confused and hurting as much as me, he didn't give up and continued to find new ways or different tactics to defeat Anna.

I thank the professional team who supported us and still do, to this day from Westmead Children's Hospital, particularly the kind and hard working Annaleise Robertson and Dr Sloane Madden.

Last, but certainly not least, I thank Summer for being a brave little girl who continues to take on the devil.

Grace X

Resources

Maudsley Family Therapy, also known as Family Based Treatment provides family therapy for the treatment of Anorexia Nervosa. It was devised by Christopher Dare and colleagues at the Maudsley Hospital in London in 1985. It is a proven treatment that is most effective in assisting patients under 18 and within 3 years of the onset of their illness.

The Maudsley approach does not view the family at fault, in fact they work with you as a family group believing that there is no better place for the child than to be home having the love and family support required to get well.

There are three phases involved in the Maudsley method.

* Weight restoration.
* Returning control over eating back to the adolescent.
* Establishing a healthy adolescent identity.

The treatment usually lasts one year and involves between 15 – 20 therapy sessions. This approach can mostly be construed as an intensive outpatient treatment where parents play an active and positive role.

Contact:

Westmead Children's Hospital, Sydney, Australia

Adolescent Medicine

Phone: (02) 9845 2446

Extra Resources

The Butterfly Foundation
www.thebutterflyfoundation.org.au

Eating Disorders Association in your state.

NSW   www.edf.org.au

VIC   www.eatingdisorders.org.au

QLD   www.eda.org.au

SA   www.communitywebs.org
NT   Association for Mental Health - (08) 8981 4128

WA   Eating Disorders Alliance - www.carersw.asn.au

TAS   www.tas.eatingdisorders.org.au

Reachout: www.reachout.com.au

For outside Australia, links can be easily found to Eating Dissorder Associations, Blogs, facebook support pages and information by completing an online search.

Please also consider seeking assistance from your Doctor or Paediatrician.

WARNING SIGNS OF *ANOREXIA*

Excessive Exercise

You panic after eating

Striving for perfection

The pursuit of control

Are you now having to lie?

FEARFUL OF FATNESS

Dramatic weight loss

When you look in the mirror are you seeing fat when in fact you are wasting away?

Monthly period stops

Rigid dieting

What does Anorexia do to your Body and mind?

Depression and Suicide

Hair Loss

Thyroid Hormone Decreases

Metabolism slows

Low white blood cell count

Heart failure and DEATH

Heart decays as body looks for protein

Slower heart rate causes - fatigue, fainting excess sleep

Rough, dry, scaly skin

Organs deteriorate

Lanugo Appearance - layer of soft down like hair all over body

Muscles waste away

Hands swell - may turn blue

Anorexia isolates you from everyone

Introduction by Babs Helleman

Babs is Head of English at The King's School in Parramatta, NSW, and a published author of a number of Secondary English textbooks.

This book reflects the reality for both the daughter, Summer and the family, who live through what can only be described as "hell" for a period of 9 months.

It is designed to help families understand how invasive the disease of Anorexia Nervosa is and how the balance between a normal, healthy life can be very fragile. Through reading Grace's diary accounts and Summer's poetic responses it is hoped that every reader will gain an insight into this disease - one that is often hidden from the public eye.

It is ironic that both the sufferer and the family see a degree of shame associated with this disease, perhaps best captured in Grace's entry of October 8th when she expresses that if it was cancer the "family could fight the battle together." It is clear, that whilst the family, with unconditional love can help, ultimately it is only Summer who can and must fight the demon in order to recover. This is why the disease is so hard for the family, who in many respects remain powerless. All logic and beliefs are challenged; all the instilled values are flaunted as the sufferer becomes consumed by an inner demon, in this text, thoughtfully named "Anna" to represent Anorexia.

The title of this text "I will not give up on my daughter" is an important mantra that gives strength to Grace and ultimately Summer. Grace's diary entries are real as is Summer's poetry. Both reflect their inner turmoil and determination, yet also reveal the devastating impact of Anorexia on the individual and the family. They capture their inner thoughts at significant times as each tries to fight the disease in particularly distinct ways.

This book is essential reading, not only for the families affected but for all teenage girls and boys. The public perception is that it is a "girls" disease but this is not the case. Dr Mark Warren from the Cleveland Centre for Eating Disorders states:

ED in men was thought to be almost non-existent, in the 80's and 90's about 10% and now 25-30%. So all we know is that it is more prevalent than was previously thought. In addition, boys engage in some behaviour unusual for girls- including steroid use, spitting, and over the counter muscle enhancers. If we include these behaviours, the prevalence of ED in boys may be even higher.

I hope this book will be read widely and taught in secondary schools as part of the Personal, Health & Development programme. It also has a place in the English classroom.

It's not the difficulties of life

that defines you,

You can't help that.

It's what you do AFTER the difficulty

that really tests who you are.

Grace
November 2012

15

Foreword

As a Counsellor, my main purpose is to listen and assist my client to arrive at their own conclusion and decision. My job is to then support and offer ways on how they will then get from point A to point B.

As a Counsellor, I was unable to help my daughter; I was far too close to the situation. I decided to drop the "professional" hat and just be her Mum, I couldn't be both.

So I now will attempt to draw from my experience and share with you my thoughts - remembering everyone is different and everyone will experience a different journey. Anorexia is such an unchartered illness (still) however - if there are just 3 things I hope you gain from reading this as a parent, caretaker or friend, these are:

1. Trust your instincts. You know your child best, if you feel Anorexia could be a factor as behaviour, mood and the weight loss is present and you are still having doubts, don't wait for this "thing" to pass, it is not a cold - it won't pass, it will take hold and get worse.

2. Get help for your child. Don't be afraid to ask for help for yourself and don't think that information will be fast coming. You really do need to find out things for yourself, ask lots of questions, read and Google, even when your loved one is under Hospital care.

3. I think this is the most important because if Anorexia doesn't kill your child, the guilt will. Be careful that you aren't a casualty of the guilt. Please believe me when I say that "you" or your "child" is NOT to blame for this illness. Anorexia does not only effect dysfunctional families, single parent families, poor families, over indulged families, low income families or high income families. Anorexia does not discriminate. This thing attacks "happy and normal"

families too. Don't waste your time trying to find blame - put your energies into fighting Anna.

If you are like me, and have other children, this is the time to be open and honest with them. Sit down together and answer any and all questions they have about Anorexia, the behavioural, psychological and physical symptoms that they are seeing, but not understanding. Even though you are in crisis mode, so are your other children. For us, we used to be a functional, happy family and had a fulfilling busy life that suddenly morphed into a dysfunctional, explosive and erratic one. Even though Summer required 24 hour care and monitoring, and you are exhausted and emotionally spent, you just have to find that bit extra for the other kids in the household. It is very hard (what an understatement) and you will ask yourself every day how you got here. Unfortunately, there is no answer other than to keep on going and brace yourself for the ride!

So much can go wrong with having Anorexia, the side effects and possible long term damage is mind blowing. The fact that your child either no longer can attend school or is failing miserably is another factor that will cause you stress, particularly if your child is in their senior years of school. My stress was through the roof and at times I couldn't remember what I had for dinner by the time I fell into bed.

I learnt very quickly to write things down that I had agreed to, for there were many times I was caught out and I'm also certain there were times I was being taken advantage of by Mia and James when it came to extra pocket money or parties that I don't remember agreeing to. What helped my family was structure, routine and keeping the household running as smoothly as possible. Maintaining as much "normal" as possible, insisting the other children maintained their sports, friendships, school responsibilities and household chores was important.

You will at times, doubt your own strength and your ability to keep going at it again and again and again, day after day after week after month and in our case, after year. You will want to give up and walk out the door yourself.

There will be times that you will prefer to take the easier option than to demand your Anorexic child to eat. Let's face it, who really wants the argument, the piercing screams, the psychotic head thrashing or the risk of her running away, or worse, hurting herself? But you can't, you just can't. Be assured, you will find out more about yourself in this time like I did. I have sacrificed so much during this time, anything from my health, my work, my friendships, my social life, my dreams, my husband and myself. I know I cannot keep doing what I am doing as I will fall apart, get sick or worse. To be a carer is very demanding, to be a carer for a child who has developed a mental illness is insufferable. You will miss and grieve for the child you once had, even though the person in front of you looks like your child, right now, she might as well be a perfect stranger.

At the back of your mind, you will always wonder what the trigger was, what happened, what was said and what caused the arrival of Anorexia? I did eventually find out.

Summer and I have been working on Book 2 whilst I was finalising this one ready for print. It is about the second year of living with Anorexia Nervosa.
Unfortunately life for us has been even more demanding, upsetting and at times impossibly overwhelming. Mia wanted to write "Jokes, wait for Book 2. Life for us is about

to get real" but thought better of it, because it isn't a game, and certainly not a topic to be taken lightly.

My family's story is not a happy one, it is challenging and very raw. I hope it brings comfort if you are going through something similar, for at least you can feel that you are not alone and that what you are experiencing is par for the course of living with Anna(rexia).

Thank you for reading our story and purchasing our book. A proportion of the proceeds will be donated to the Children's Hospital to assist with the research and treatment of Eating Disorders.

I would now like to introduce you to my family.
My husband Derek
My eldest daughter Mia
Summer, the co-author of this book
and my
youngest son, James

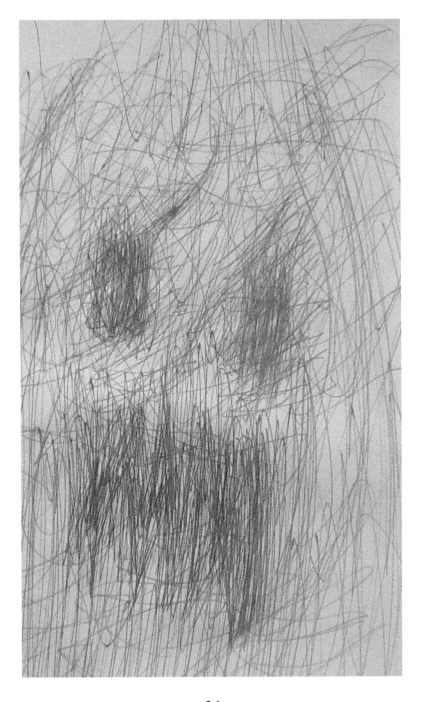

24

Letting Anorexia in is
the Biggest Mistake of My Life

Have you ever felt like
you were being controlled?

Have you ever felt you were possessed
by a thought you can't remember?

Have you ever been told by other people
that this isn't normal?

Have you realised you have an utter obsession
with something that you loathe?

Well that's what it feels like living
with Anna(rexia).

It all started with a comment,
A comment that has stuck with me

my whole life,

By someone that I didn't think I would remember
after all these years.

But that comment, has changed my life.
That comment will make me stronger
when I finally get through this journey of
inner strength and self discovery.

Those words, fat, big, weight and kilogram.
The words don't scare me,
It's the meaning of the word,
I was and am avoiding.
I created a game.
A game of hunger.
A game of pain

A game that caused me to lose my laugh.

Disappointment is all I feel

When I look back and remember

My decision to join the game of anorexia.

I lost myself.

I lost Summer.

This is my story of how I will

get her back.

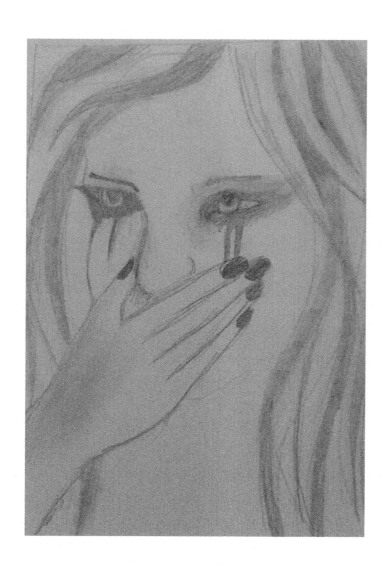

How it all Began

We have a new word that is very disliked in my home at the moment - disliked is probably not strong enough for the damage it's doing to my family - when my girls were younger and experimenting with the English language their most hated sounding words were bra, ulcer, period - well today we added a new one - anorexia nervosa.

How could this be happening to my bright, funny, smart, slim, healthy, high self esteemed, little 13 year old daughter? Her eating habits changed about 45 days ago - when she began to bring her lunch home uneaten – her explanation was that she was too busy at lunchtime and that none of her friends really ate lunch - we compromised and I suggested she take food that she could eat and walk with, after all that's what teenagers do - walk and cruise around the school grounds - so in her lunch bag went 2 pieces of fruit and a salada with cheese and Vegemite. This all came home too - in fact she was trying to skip breakfast, afternoon tea and expect that I would be happy with her decision for a massively reduced dinner. Reality hit when I raised the issue with the school and they phoned me back requesting a meeting with my husband and I for the next afternoon.

After a long introduction of how our daughter is a fabulous student, well liked and has settled into her new school beautifully, we are hit with the statement, "but we think she has the beginnings of anorexia nervosa!"

Hang on a minute I remember saying, we are here about the kids of year 8 not eating their lunches - why are you saying that we are getting close to Summer going down the eating disorder trail?

Eating disorder - what does that mean?

Does it mean a kid who is just off food right now?

Is it just that she's too busy to be interested in food?

What the...?

Are we talking about the same person here - surely you are joking right?

The school bell sounded and our meeting was quickly wrapped up. A phone number to a local known counsellor was handed to us.

"Good luck, we are here if you need us during the school holidays."

(June/ July school holidays – duration 3 weeks)

Derek and I stood in the school playground waiting for Summer and James to walk up and meet us. It was like I was standing in the middle of a vortex, suddenly quiet, yet activity and noise was apparently all around us. My world, and life as I knew it, stopped at that point.

Now here comes the denial part, it only lasted for a few minutes, but it went a little like this. Okay this can be fixed over the break right? Summer will be home and can eat lunch with me and we can do some baking and go out for dinner as a family, do fun activities and surely that will take her mind off all of this. Perhaps whilst we are at it, let's take the kids skiing for a week to get away and take in the mountain air - a good break from routine and everything will just return to normal, right?

It was now time for Derek and I to have a talk with Summer.

Anger was certainly the emotion that stands out for me most that day coming home from Summer's school. Rage - I was fuming at Summer - how could she have achieved so much and become so hooked on losing weight??

How ridiculous - just stop it now I growled at her. Do as you're told, I'm your Mother and you will do as I say regarding this and I will not accept this behaviour from you!

Pfft – you're right ! What was I thinking?

My husband Derek, calmly said to me that perhaps I should take a minute as I was irrational, angry, emotional and definitely having an almighty Mother of a melt down. "FINE" I said, and took the dog for a walk and kept my distance so I could get my head around it all.

Panic

Our job is to guide and gently steer them to try new things and find passion in what they like. School is important but not the only lessons available in life - our home is always open to the children's friends, we do the birthday parties, we do the animals - dog, cat, guinea pigs, rabbits, ducks and now we have 3 chooks who come into the house to say hello if the door gets left open - corny I know but they are named Butter, Sweet and Sour.

We do the big family vacations, camping, skiing, Fiji, a 10 day Pacific Cruise, day trips, overnight trips and weekends away. Perhaps Hawaii this year as James is older and much more capable of traveling longer distances and is at the age to remembr the trip. We do it all - we love our family, the bond we have, the sharing of ourselves and the immense fun we all have - we enjoy our children and they get a good laugh on our account too - they really do know we are doing the best we can .

So what did I do first? I contacted the Counsellor to make an appointment. I needed advice, information... SOMETHING...ANYTHING to make sense of all of this. I had an appointment already with my Doctor for two days time, so I decided to wait until then.

So for me, I couldn't sleep that night, I cried and cried and cried until no more tears would come. I headed for my home office with a cup of tea and began to Google Anorexia Nervosa - What is it? How do you get it? The cure? What help is there available? Books to read? Then I found the site where parents and the sufferers themselves had written and shared their stories - pictures, images, ads, slogans, I was in information overload, but I needed and required more and more information .

By 7 am, when the house was waking up I had come full circle from feeling intense anger to being a calmer, more ordered thinker. I knew I needed to be there for Summer more than ever, and I wanted to be. What do you do when you are presented with this - panic certainly and suggest eating would be good start - how about the absurdity of it all, after all, aren't we the family who has three great kids, me who decided to give up my career and become a stay at home Mum, a Dad who worked hard in our own business and provided a great life for all of us, our kids who are great at school, happy, creative, sporty, respectful and that the 5 of us just love hanging out together. We are the quintessential family who have dinner together, who have an on going yearly point scoring game of UNO, where Dad and son have found dirt bike riding for their common ground to have fun, communicate man stuff, relax and to bond. We encourage, support, love and advocate there is no such word as can't.

I had to be the one she turned to - to cuddle her, to not judge her, to love her unconditionally.

I am her Mum.

I

will

not

give

up

on

my

daughter.

Get a Grip

Do Something

I went to my Doctor's appointment that I had arranged a couple of weeks prior as I had some health issues.

Whilst there, I raised my concerns of Summer and began telling her about the past few days in a non logical manner. I poured out a series of concerns which had my Doctor shift gear and pay very close attention to me. We made an appointment for the following day to bring Summer in for a check up.

I felt deceitful when I got home and told Summer I had made a Doctor's appointment for her as she had been complaining of a sore throat.

Reality Check

Whilst Summer and I were in the Doctor's waiting room, I asked Summer if she wanted me to come into the Doctor's room with her. In one giant shift of behaviour, so totally out of character, Summer stood up and refused to be there with the full intention of walking out. Clearly the penny had dropped that we were there for something other than her sore throat!

(I'm glad I had geared the Doctor up, for she was well prepared to ask other key questions after attending to the business of the sore throat.)

The appointment was all about Summer, she could do all the talking. I stayed quiet whilst the Doctor asked questions and did a basic health check. "It appears you don't like food that much Summer? Perhaps your low mood is a result of that too? I'm concerned about your hands being blue and that your energy levels are really down."

Around then, I interjected with "is this all related to the sore throat? A virus of some sort? Can you also please check Summer's temperature, not for a fever, but that she is cold and I'm concerned about the bruises that seem to appear for no reason on her legs and arms."

Now I have never been a good actor, the plot was blown wide open and Summer was now feeling she was backed into a corner and started to get agitated and angry. Again, so totally out of character!

The appointment was wrapped up after an hour, and we were sent off to get some blood tests and an ECG. Summer's heart rate had dropped to 45 b.p.m. Which had us already in a dangerous state, as the heart rate drops further when we rest and are sleeping.

We, however, were not aware of the dangers - Summer was very upset getting her blood taken, she has had blood taken and needles before, but her smart mouth to the Pathologist and her un-cooperative behaviour had my alarm bells ringing off the hook.

Summer's weight and height were also taken. The Pathologist was inexperienced and didn't pick up on the fact that a 13 year old was undergoing these types of tests, so she was ridiculously jolly and attempting to crack jokes - all of which were wasted on a demonically moody child and a fretful Mother.

Summer and I returned home 4 hours after our scheduled 9:30am appointment emotionally exhausted.

Thank goodness Derek was home.

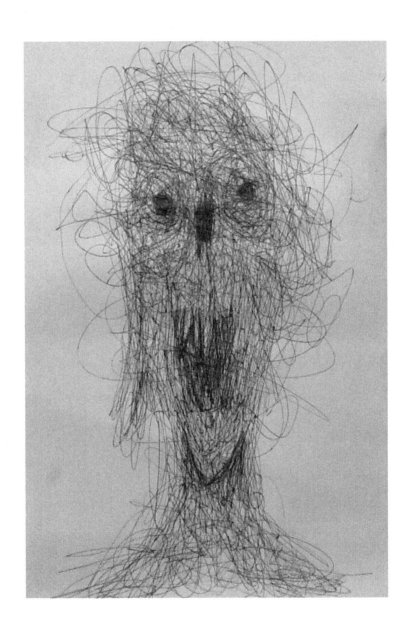

Summer Speaks from the Heart

She is Coming

It's almost like you are drowning,

You have a choice

Stay under or swim to the surface.

Anna told me to stay under,

She is forceful,

She is mean,

She will tell you lies.

She told me not to eat.

She re-wires your thoughts

Replaces the real you with a new picture

One you will replicate

No matter what it takes.

The more engrossed you become.

It is normal.

The constant black cloud hovers

Not because I let it,

But because I couldn't stop it!

I had no control over Anna.

I wasn't happy,

I was cold,

I didn't smile or laugh,

I didn't eat,

I didn't drink unless forced.

She was in control.

I had opened the door to a stranger,

And she consumed me.

At first I cut out junk food and then lunch by a quarter, then by half, then three quarters. I decided to hide the last quarter in my gums and spit it out when I went to brush my teeth. I did eat dinner just to stop me from fainting.

The volume of food wasn't even close enough to keep my bones from showing and my skin from bruising.

I felt guilty when I ate so I ran up and down the hill at my school to burn extra fat that Anna told me I had. Eventually I became so disgusted at the thought of food that I fought with my parents. I thought food was unnatural and I became obsessed.

As Anna grew in strength I became physically smaller, so small that there wasn't enough of me to keep me warm, to keep me happy, not even enough to keep my heart beating or my mouth breathing.

I lost memory and concentration, Anna was making me eat myself from inside out.

Even now I forget what I'm doing because I left a gap for Anna to creep in to send me backwards and against my family.

I
want
help

I

need

help

I

have

Help

Dad's Take

Here am I sitting on golden sands as the sun peaks over the horizon of Merimbula beach. The start of our summer holiday. The start of a new year. Looking forward. Looking back. What a year it has been.

I've always been a person who sees their glass as half full, never half empty, but Summer's illness certainly put that theory to the test. I would love to think that I have a special relationship with my children. I love them all individually, dearly...

My story begins in the middle of May.
Summer was born on my birthday back in February 1999. For whatever reason Summer and I have always had a sort of

kinship. As a Father and for any Father reading this, we all hold our daughters dearly, do we not?

Summer was in the kitchen one weekend baking muffins as she does and stuffing them into her face as fast as she could ice them. The following weekend baking away as she does, but this time she wouldn't touch them. This was only the beginning. It was as quick as a light turning on and off, blink and you're there.

I spent many an hour researching and talking with Summer about the amount of food required for the body to breath in and out. Approximately 2,000 calories per day and that's just sitting on the lounge being a sloth.

All this was to no avail. Grace, my lovely wife, who was ever vigilant, took Summer to her Doctor. Summer's heart rate was 45 BPM. Being totally devoid of any knowledge; we put our faith in the GP that all was okay except that Summer's weight and temperature was down. Permission was given by our GP to take that family holiday, so off we went to the snow.

Summer came to me on the first day absolutely frozen and in tears. She was so cold, her hands, feet and face were frozen. Every extremity, just like ice. I set about finding whatever measures possible to warm her.

On the drive back to our accommodation, Summer fell asleep in the front seat with the heater full on, when we arrived, Summer wouldn't wake, my heart was tearing apart, what if...

Thank God it wasn't the case.

Introducing *Mia*

I'm a classic 15 year old, I like to eat, sleep, and sleep some more.

I have 2 siblings who have their good and bad days.

I have a Mum who now kills down any argument that arises so as to keep the peace.

I have a Dad who just irritates me, don't get me wrong, our father/daughter relationship is great. It's just that he's a Dad and "Dads are supposed to be annoying"!

Where do I fit in?

I'm Mia.

I rule the roost of the little people and I'm the one with the hardest punch.

At the beginning of the year, things were going great, just peachy.

I thought this

was my year.

I was unstoppable,

unbreakable even.

But things change,

and boy,

did they ever!

Time To Get Away?

Summer and I returned to the Doctor to discuss the results of the tests. Underweight for age, low BMI %, dehydrated, low heart rate, low body temperature, bloods all fine, but the cessation of Summer's periods were a concern.

I did ask the question of my Doctor about going to the snow, questioning whether it was a wise decision, but think about our plan?

family time

a break away

fresh mountain air.

healthy, happy, fun

a fabulous idea quite frankly, agreed by all

this was a good idea!

So we went to the snow for our annual family ski trip.

Isn't hindsight a wonderful thing! The signs were all there! Summer was tired, hard to wake and feeling the cold more than her 9 year old brother. Instead we dressed her in triple clothing, ensured she had all the right snow gear and stopped and rested her every hour. Summer insisted she was fine and didn't want to go back to the Hotel, yet she still struggled. On the second day, her toes and fingers were blue and she couldn't warm up. The pain she was feeling was so intense that she began to shake and scream. Okay, time to go home!

School holidays proved to be a real shake down - I went back to basics and got all the baby books out to re think a basic menu plan and to encourage eating smaller amounts but every couple of hours.

As a Mum our job is to nurture, feed, love, ensure health, wellbeing and offer a calm, stable, comfortable, safe and loving home environment.

All possible until anorexia came to live with us.

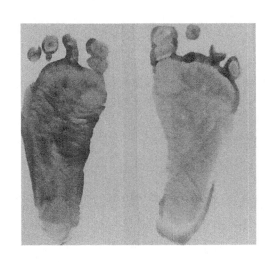

Baby Steps

We have come up with a plan... A plan to take baby steps!
A plan to make the numbers go up! Even if it's minimal, it's
still up, and up is forward and forward is normal.

I don't want to see my body change,

get bigger,

get uglier,

get fat ...

That's a scary thing,

Being so afraid of something

So easy.

Something so simple!

But in the head space I'm in right now,

It's how I feel.

57

Mia Talks About Anna(Rexia)

Look who got the incredibly horrible, life changing and idiotic bug called Anorexia?

It wasn't me

It wasn't my parents - thank God

It wasn't my brother

It wasn't my dog, cat, fish, chickens or any other animal that we have.

Nah! It was my sister.

My 13 year old baby sister.

She is starving herself to death basically.

The fact that my sister thought she was fat and ugly was confusing and irritating enough - the fights that came from Anorexia were huge!

I felt like a Gladiator who would, or at times, should have, charged through the room and slashed us all down having realised there was an actual battle that needed to be fought.

Anorexia was horrific; add in the Doctors and Therapists and you unleash a time bomb.

Being the older Sister, you feel some kind of responsibility for what happens to your younger siblings.

Example:
"Mia, Mia! That guy cheated on me!" She would say. "Right, where is that *@$?@#*? I'm gunna smash his head off his neck" I would say.

OR

"Mia! I tripped and scraped my leg! Help me stop the waterfall of blood leaking out!" She would say. "Here's a towel!" I would say.

You get my drift, being older, more responsibility ...

Blah Blah Blah!

So you can only imagine what position I was in when my sister got herself into this... PREDICAMENT.

To give you an idea, it was like pressing the shut down button on the computer, pulling the power cord, punching through the screen, snapping the memory card and throwing the whole thing in the garbage.

Total and utter lock down -

I didn't want to hear about it!

Basically, I wanted to remove myself totally from it and just continue on with my life.

But was life that fair?

NO

It pushed and pulled in places we didn't want to be pushed and pulled and now we have experienced this ..."thing".

I

I

am

concerned

that

it

will

always

be

in

our

lives

and

we

will

have

to

get

used

to

it

just

floating

around.

The Eye of the Storm

Life has been very difficult. Summer is still refusing to eat. Her temper is hideous and unnerving. Mia and James are finding her intolerable and my gorgeous family is imploding. Derek and I are scrambling for answers; we are now seeing the Counsellor recommended by the school.

The Counsellor is a one hour drive away, she had a daughter who suffered from Anorexia and certainly had a lot to say. Summer would go into her office and then maybe an hour later I would be invited in for the attack on how I could do better to make poor Summer's life more bearable. Are you kidding me? The Counsellor was helpful to Summer, but also did a very good job in undermining the parents authority. The Counsellor was looking for the reason as to why we were in this mess. I must admit, I had never known anyone or experienced anything pertaining to Anorexia Nervosa so I was flying blind. This prompted me to look closer to the reason Summer developed Anorexia, but it was clear that she was turning away from Derek and I and we had no hope in getting through to her let alone getting her to eat.

Summer continued to lose weight, she fainted at school, she was freezing and would come home from school and take a long hot bath. She continued on her appeal that she wasn't feeling well and therefore had no appetite. She ran away a couple of times, in spite, as we were telling her to come to the table for dinner. Summer continued exercising, she was so weakened now that we had no choice but to pull her out of her soccer team, tell her school she could not engage in physical activity and after another fainting episode we kept her home from school.

Remember, at this point we had not had a confirmed diagnosis of Anorexia Nervosa, though we clearly suspected it was the case. Basically, Derek and I were going from the advice from books, our local G.P. and the Counsellor.

We felt backed into a corner, so our next step was to phone the hospital directly to get some advice, help, direction ... Anything.

On our last visit with the Counsellor and before we begged the hospital to assist, her parting words were a definite warning that Anorexia can lead to Bulimia and that my heart would be broken many, many times.

You can live for a month without food but only a week without water.

Thank goodness for Derek's persuasiveness, we had an in road to the hospital.

Facts

1 person in every 1,000 will develop anorexia nervosa.

1 person out of every 10 with anorexia will die.

In every 10 people with an eating disorder, 2 will be male.

More people die of an eating disorder each year than people with a smoking related disease.

95% of those who have eating disorders are between the ages of 12 and 25.

The cost of treatment of an eating disorder in the United States ranges from $500-$2,000 per day. The average cost for a month of inpatient treatment is $30,000. It is estimated that individuals with eating disorders need anywhere from 3 - 6 months of inpatient care.

In 2012 more than 913,000 people in Australia suffered from eating disorders. The total socio economic cost of eating disorders in 2012 for Australia was $69.7 billion.

Dad's Take

When we arrived home from our snow trip, I was hoping that I could put a scare into Summer with a reality check. I called the intake nurse at Westmead Children's Hospital to get the low down on what hospital life was like for Anorexic patients.

Well didn't that make heads spin! After telling the Nurse what Summer's weight and BPM were, alarm bells instantly rang. Get her in NOW! Our new contact and her team called 4 times over the next 2 hours. This was an emergency. We didn't know that our little princess could have had a heart attack, stroke or worse, died in her sleep at any time.

My heart sank. I was always told as a child that boys shouldn't cry, but my heart and soul were being torn apart as my wife drove Summer to the hospital that night.

For many a month after that I had a re-occurring dream that I was rocking Summer's frail body in my arms and telling her that it was okay to go. Even now as I type, this memory to me is very raw.

The Hospital Experience

It was Tuesday, my second school day of Term 3. I was sitting in the sun at my sister's school, it was parent teacher night. It was the night, it happened.

My body went into shock. I saw my Dad's face after a particular phone call, that's when I knew I'd taken it too far. I saw him walk over to Mum with his face locked on the ground beneath him.

The world we all knew was crumbling around us.
I knew exactly what the news was before it touched my ears.

It was time for me to go to hospital.

Leaving

I sat in silence.

Oblivious to the suroundings.

Contemplating all options.

But there were no options.

There was only one.

Leaving.

Mum packed my bag, I waved goodbye to the home I knew and was now expected to accept the unknown. I had to say goodbye to 3 of my 4 best friends. It was one of the hardest things I have ever had to do. Especially when I had no choice.

We drove, parked, walked, waited and straight after that...
Emergency Ward.

I was on a heart monitor. It was obvious to the nurses I wouldn't be leaving anytime soon.
Suddenly a nurse appeared, we were taken into a separate room. A room where they shut and locked the door! She held up a tube. A tube that was to be fed through my nose

via the back of my throat to the pit of my stomach. That was how I was to be fed.

It was almost midnight when I was transferred to a heart ward called Edgar Stephan's.

Nightmares

They made me eat.

They made me drink.

They made me sit.

I wasn't living.

I was getting help.

I didn't want.

Which made it worse.

It was in that ward where I met a beautiful girl named Claire. She kept me company during the day. We talked. We got to know each other. We also went to hospital school together.

But hospital is hospital. Whether you have a friend or not, it doesn't alter your perception of a living hell. One week had passed and it was time for me to move wards.

I was transferred to Wade Ward.
The hospital ward for eating disorders.

All the girls were so skinny. I didn't fit in at all. But yet, we were all here for the same reason. I also realised when I got there they were all obsessed. They were all extreme. But that was when I realised ... I was the same.

Deceit

I learnt their tricks.
I became one of them.
I was, one of them.
I hid food as they did.
I exercised, as they did.
I did as they did.

Only now I realise everything they had done
and continued to do
helped Anna, not me.

71

Captivity

Another week passed.

Watching, waiting, dreading.

It was meal time.

The sound of the food trolleys.

Made all of our heads spin.

Our stomachs knot.

Supervised eating.

Six times a day.

Breakfast.

Morning Tea.

Lunch.

Afternoon tea.

Dinner.

Supper.

These were the times.

We thought of escape.

We were spiteful and deceitful.

We wanted to take vengeance.

We wanted our lives back.

I wanted to go home.

It was then I was allowed a gate pass for the upcoming weekend. I could go home Friday and return to the hospital Sunday night. I could sleep in my own bed. Most important of all, eat without supervision.

I packed my bags, threw them on top of my hospital bed and watched the clock count down the hours, minutes and seconds until I would see my Dad open the door and take me home. I was happy up until I unlocked the front door of my house.

Stranger

I felt like a stranger.

Everyone looked at me differently.

It was like I wasn't welcome.

This was my house.

This wasn't my home.

My gate pass ended.

Disappointment.

So I started to enjoy hospital. It was there and only there that I felt at home. I was learning to love it. I learnt all of the

Nurses names like they were our guardians. The girls treated each other like sisters. We walked to school like friends. It was what I knew. Hospital was easier than home.

Acceptance

It's hard to think that way.

It hurts to think that way.

But it's the way we all thought.

It was my way of thinking.

I wasn't alone.

I was accepted.

Hospital was the place.

Where I wasn't different.

Hospital was hell no longer.

It was where I wanted to be.

Either way, they were the ones that made me eat.

No matter how cozy I felt, in an ironic twist I needed to go home so that I could reduce the volume of food I had to consume.

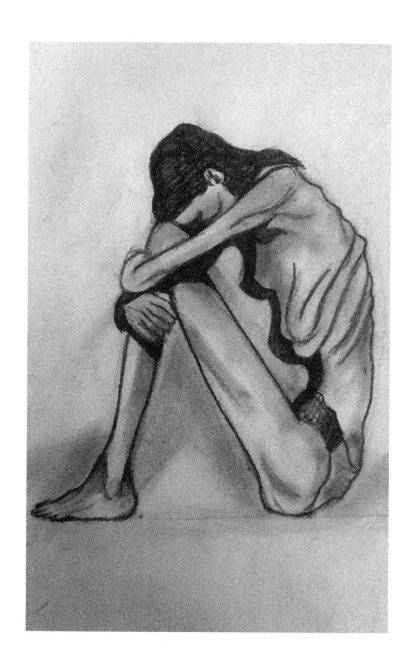

Diary extract by Grace

July 17th (7pm)

Committed and Admitted

I packed an overnight bag and took Summer to Emergency at Westmead Children's Hospital - I held Summer's hand and cried all the way whilst driving her to the hospital.

They were waiting for us, VIP'S in Emergency - the other poor people waiting way before we got there were probably wondering why we were so special - 5 minutes after arriving we were in triage, through the double doors and Summer was in a bed... taking a total of 15 minutes. A heart monitor was set up, weight taken, temperature taken, bloods taken ...

Then a feeding tube ... "Hold my hand Summer whilst the Nurses thread a tube up your nose, through the back of your mouth, down your throat right into the pit of your stomach.

"Oh and by the way Grace, if your daughter refuses any food from now on, she will have to drink it via this feeding system."

Around midnight we were transferred to the Heart Ward. The hospital is very parent friendly with roll out beds (most uncomfortable) however, it allows you to stay no matter the condition.

It's dire, but no one complains. The parents scattered around these children's wards are the heroes of life, facing the ongoing daily struggles of ordinary people in extraordinary circumstances, full of hope, kindness and positive affirmations for their child or for the parent who has entered the ward during the middle of the night.

"You are so under weight; we need to feed you whilst you are sleeping. "A bag of nutrients is hooked up overnight, a machine that beeped loudly in the quiet ward echoed through my hurting brain, a rhythm of the heart monitor, beep beep beep ... Beeeeeeep ... then alarmed if the irregular heart rate dropped below a specified number, on and on and on... I lay there watching the numbers shift on my baby daughter's heart monitor - 45, 47, 49, 44 beep beep beep !!!!

Summer was exhausted after fighting with the Nurses and Doctor in Emergency - my girl made it hard for the hospital staff. There was lots of talking and lots of reassuring, lots of hugging, hand holding, lots of I love you and it will be okay, patting her hair, helping her fall asleep.

Shhhh go to sleep

Tomorrow is a new day my darling

the

worst

is

behind

us.

The Day After

Another indication that Summer was not herself, was when the Psych team and their entourage arrived the following morning to have a chat. The senior Doctor began asking Summer questions and challenged her about her eating behaviour. Summer responded with a quick retort and asked if he was qualified and what if anything did he know about what she was going through.

The Heart Ward Had Strict Rules

Summer was eating, co-operating, resting and getting stronger - but her inner spirit was not fighting to get better and come home. Her fight was against the staff - who she believed constantly punished her by making her eat breakfast, morning tea, lunch, afternoon tea, dinner and supper.

I know we were in the heart ward, but Summer was supervised when she ate, had to ask permission to use the bathroom, couldn't get out of bed 30 minutes after a meal, was confined to a wheelchair, was not allowed visitors apart from immediate family and was not allowed to leave anything uneaten on her tray. Summer was still being fed through the tube at night, infact she preferred it to eating normally. When the time came for it to be removed, Summer was very upset. Her psychologist was called to convince her that this was the better alternative. She took a lot of convincing.

The Nurses were getting tougher, the rules more rigid and the reality of this nightmare .... was becoming clear.

The heart ward

was a holiday camp

compared

to the

eating disorder ward.

Summer's Okay

Seven days later, Summer was declared physically stable and allowed out of bed. Wheelchairs, heart monitors, tubes, wires and drips - gone ... Improvement right?

Summer was now strong enough to attend the hospital school. She could join in on some of the fun group activities that the hospital offers in the afternoon with other teen-agers. With this and a healthy eating regime in place, it was a definite start to rebuilding Summer's malnourished, tiny body.

Colour had returned to Summer's beautiful face, the gauntness, the skeletal features seemed to be disappearing, she had volume in her voice, if you were lucky you might even hear a little giggle to one of Dad's sick jokes - we were hopeful that this scare would get her back on track. Summer had gained 2.5 kilograms - we were out of danger now ... right??

Dad's Take

Westmead Children's Hospital and staff were fantastic to say the least, very tough, but very caring both to patient and parent alike.

On one occasion I spent with Summer in hospital we went to the cafeteria for dinner, Anna came too.

As much as Summer declared she was on the mend, Anna had different ideas and had Summer hiding her mash potato and whatever else she could, under her schnitzel crumbs. Dinner came to a crashing end.

Facts

There is no one cause for the onset of anorexia nervosa eating disorder.

Predisposing factors, including genetic susceptibility, have been shown in research to account for up 60% of cause of onset.

Precipitating factors are often related to emotional factors and stressors including trauma.

Social and media expectations also receive some blame.

Short answer: a combination of biology and environment.

Learning Tricks

One of my and Derek's biggest concerns before Summer was transferred from the heart ward to the eating disorder ward was the additional information she was about to see, experience, learn, and be taught.

You have heard cases where criminals who go into jail come out more skilled in illegal activities. Well my little girl, who thought dieting and getting slim could be done without eating, learnt very creative ways to survive in the ward.

Girls would paint their finger nails so they could hide the butter or vegemite under their finger nails to avoid putting it on their toast. Hide food in their gums, because Nurses checked their mouths - but not above their teeth and even take the sterile gloves and fill them with food then throw the package out the window when opportunity arose. The girls were always watched, yet they managed to steal the Nurses roster, photocopy it at the hospital school – tape it under a table then when the shift hand over occurred and the Nurses were briefly meeting and exchanging information - this was the time for purging. So be it, if they had to wait until 2 am in the morning!

As you can imagine we loved the fact that a 16 year old girl advised Summer that the best form of exercise and the most successful way to burn off calories is of course to have sex with anyone who is willing!

Drinking a litre of water before weigh in will ensure success and allow you to go home, wearing double the clothing also helps. The same young lady advising the sex exercise theory was also the same girl who had snuck 4 bottles of fat burning tablets in on readmission! So now, our once innocent, sweet 13 year old daughter knew about diuretics, irresponsible sex, hiding food, throwing up and how to deceive your parents about how much food you have eaten.

Water

loading

and

filling pockets

with rocks

at weigh in

came later.

Facts

Question: What should I do if I think someone has anorexia?

If you suspect someone you know has anorexia, it is important to express your concerns to them. Approach them in a compassionate and nonjudgmental manner. They may become angry and defensive. Don't give up. It may take time before they are ready to open up. Tell them you are concerned about their health.
Do not comment on how they look. Avoid placing blame, shame, or guilt.

Encourage them to seek help from a parent, school counsellor, Doctor or any adult they trust.

Dad's Take

To think anorexia was just a teenage fad to lose some weight, or even worse a school yard bully, think again, this is your worst nightmare!

To even think that your child has been taken over by a demon is ridiculous. Well hold onto your seats, you, your family and your child are in for one hell of a ride.

Possessed would become closer to the truth than you think. With rapid weight loss, the brain shrinks, as a result, clarity of thought and the normal ability to process information or reason is thrown out the window. The brain is one of the last elements to return. Seeing Summer in hospital was tough, heart monitor, feeding tube, thin, frail, eyes that looked huge compared to her small face, and her skin was the colour grey.

Grace and I took it in turns to spend the night on uncomfortable fold out lounges, but we knew this was the best place for Summer right now.

Mia's Definition

of Anorexia Nervosa

Emotions are only chemicals that run through your brain, making you react to situations in different personas.

True

The non infectious disease, Anorexia, is an attack on the brains thought patterns, making a person fear fat and forcing themselves into starvation.

True

These definitions capture the effects of anorexia.

True

The Hospital, Counsellors, Doctors and Nurses explain Anorexia. Hey, they even give you a handbook called "Handling Your Stupid Emotions While Starving Yourself".

False

No, there's only a certain amount of what Google definitions can give to you.

Taking these definitions and trying to fit them into your life is like sticking both your hands in your mouth and realising just one is difficult. Wrapping your head around Anorexia is hard enough, never mind all the emotions that tumble after it.

You see and experience things you never thought you would. You feel stuff that can put you in an off mood for weeks.

You definitely take a good look at yourself,

find your weaknesses,

your strengths

and

you learn how to build them up

and

break them down.

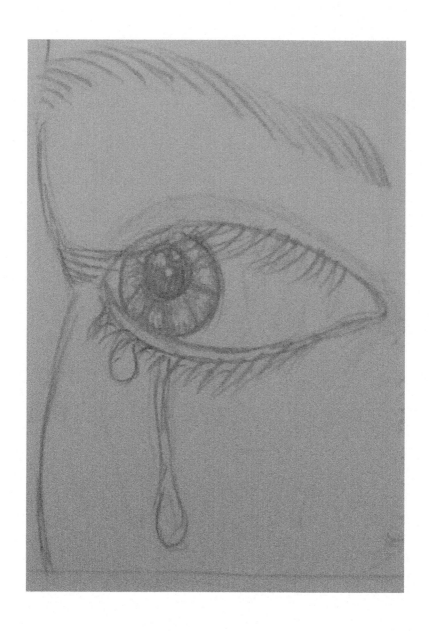

97

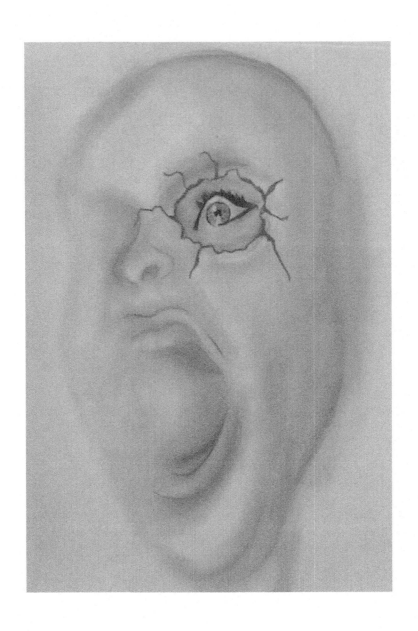

Strategies

It's come back...

Stronger, smarter and harder.

But this time, there are different words

speaking to me.

A demand

An order

She is telling me that my only choice is bulimia.

Making myself sick.

I'm sick of fighting. I'm tired of people treating me

differently.

I have fought and fought with Anna until I thought she

had given up trying to destroy me.

I was wrong ... again.

I don't think I have any fight left in me to keep going.

Anna

What if she never goes.

What if this happens forever.

What if my only option

Is death.

I can't handle it.

I want to go.

I need to go.

But I can't go.

That's what hurts me most,

The fact that,

If I do go,

It will hurt my family more,

They would have travelled

This not yet finished path

For nothing.

I need my parents to be my friends, my teachers to be my guardians and my brother and sister to be my supporters.

Anna 2

I will and I am

Trying my best

To push Anna as far away

As possible.

It really is like a never ending phone call

From someone that broke you.

Someone that you USED to trust.

You can either answer it.

Or ignore it.

And then there is me.

I'm just standing in one spot,

Letting it ring.

An easy decision,

But a hard action

To follow through.

Almost impossible.

A Trial Visit

Eating Disorders rob you blind - they steal from you whilst you're not watching. They change personalities that were once vivacious, cheeky, fun and energetic to morose, dark, almost psychotic, argumentative, depressed, irrational and unpredictable. My Summer had changed for sure, growing up almost overnight, a knowledge base far beyond her years. I kept repeating to the family how she had changed, no one could see it - but I could.

Our aim now was to get her out of the disorder ward and back home where surely we could make a difference. We pushed for this. After all, we could look after her, re-program her thoughts, nurture, feed, restore her to her former self? Love conquers all? Right?

After a family therapy session to assess if we were a "fit" family to have Summer come home 10 days early from her anticipated release date - we passed and were allowed to bring Summer home for an overnight trial visit. This trial occurred twice before she was allowed to return home full time.

We were pleased she was home, our family of 5 was back together again. We were all exhausted, we got in late evening and I rustled up a quick basic dinner for all of us ...

Mistake number 1

Whilst 4 out of 5 were grateful for something to eat, Summer was unimpressed.

This was really hard for her as she had now been away from home for 3 weeks. Summer now felt like an intruder and that she didn't belong here at home. That night Summer ran away, she scarred us all.
Adjusting back into the fragile, tired, family home was more difficult than we anticipated.

Summer tells how it is

Being Me

None of them get it.

None of them know how hard it is

To fight a mental battle.

With thoughts

You are so used to thinking.

It's confusing,

Telling myself to stop thinking inwardly.

It's not a voice speaking to me,

Telling me what to do.

It's more like a negative

And positive voice arguing.

But I can't tell which one is Anna

And which one is me.

But clearly everyone else seems to know.

Explaining

anorexia

to

someone

is

like

saying

to

them

hold

your

breath

until

your

head

hurts.

Harder than it sounds!

Almost impossible.

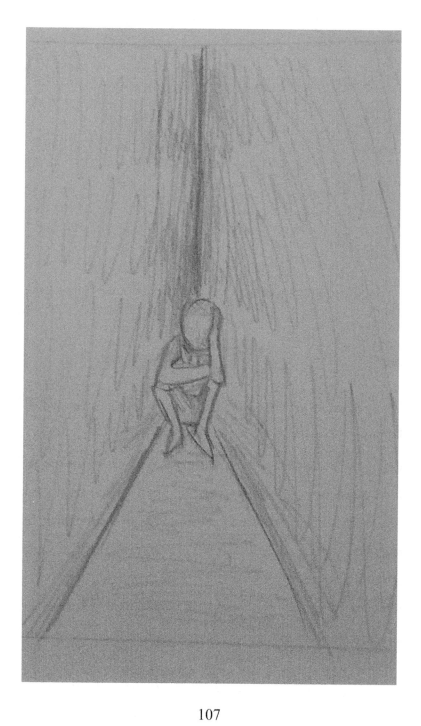

107

Dad's Take

Soon enough it was time for Summer to come home...

Supervised Eating

One particular evening that I will never forget is one when Summer refused to eat the last little bit on her plate. Grace took Mia and James to bed whilst I stayed with Summer at the dining table. To see my child one minute screaming her lungs out at me, then the next crumpled up on the floor in tears was just heart breaking to say the least. But you must stay the course.

Many a meal time was spent in anger with Summer or should I say Summer spent many a meal time in anger with Grace and I.

People, even more than things,

have to be

restored

renewed

revived

reclaimed

and redeemed

never throw out anyone.

Audrey Hepburn

Mia Reflects on when

Summer came Home

So to set the scene for you, Summer had just returned from hospital, after being nearly dead and clearly still mentally unstable. Family therapy sessions had just started.

For the time Summer was away, it was kind of nice in a way (I'm trying to say this without sounding like a complete uncaring and selfish @&¢$#¥) so stay with me.

Being in a household for 3 months with constant fighting and always turning up to school with a frown on my face was beginning to be sort of a letdown. So when the fighting and frowning went away for nearly 4 weeks, you could imagine how great it felt to have things liven up a bit.

So when Summer came back, even though we visited her in Hospital, we kind of backed off - like meeting a stranger for the first time and keeping only to the basics in conversation. I understand how she may have felt lonely, but words can't describe how breakable everything was. Our family was just holding it together by a string and Summer was holding the scissors.

It took a fabulous one day, until the fights began - wanna guess what they were about? It starts with "F" and you can EAT it.

At that time, all I felt was anger towards Summer and this situation.

Anger is an awful feeling, it doesn't seem to have a limit, and it just grows.

I stopped crying about the whole anorexia thing when Summer first went to hospital. Initially, I did it because I didn't want Mum to feel more horrible, but really it was because I blamed Summer for tearing our family apart in the worst way possible.

Trust and Trusted

What is trust?

What do you do with it?

Who do you give it to?

Choose wisely.

Trust has to be earned.

Trust is like a piece of paper.

Once it's crumpled,

It will never be perfect.

My parents and I have a relationship

Based on two key factors,

Love and trust.

The sad thing is,

There is no trust.

They both expect me to trust them,

Trust them with what?

Trust them with my life,

With my teddy?

No - they want me to invest

All of my trust in them,

Yet I see them both

As strangers.

Trust is a two way street.

I don't expect them to trust me,

But when I'm telling them the truth

I expect them to trust me -

Yet they eat up my heart.

That hurts.

The two people

Who are the closest to me

Are the ones hurting me the most.

I don't trust them.

I love them with all of my heart,

But I don't trust them,

Because they don't trust me.

Trust has to be earned.

Only I know the truth,

Only I know how I feel.

But I don't want to be alone

In these truthful words.

I wish I could record my thoughts

And play them back.

To prove that I AM trustworthy.

I am moving forward.

My parents are holding me back.

Telling me what to do,

I take a step back.

Am I the only one

That still believes in Santa

Or the Easter Bunny?

I believe in the impossible.

I believe in magic and spirits.

Reincarnation.

Something after death.

Second chances.

I am a believer.

I trust in my beliefs.

But there are people

Who don't have my trust

And don't deserve to be believed.

I don't lie.

I haven't lied about food for a long time.

But yet my words aren't enough to persuade the

unpersuaded.

Direct them to the truth that is ringing in their ears,

But yet goes unrecognised.

My heart is fragile,

It breaks easily.

My heart broke tonight.

It still aches.

The pain is intense

It has numbed my head, heart and soul.

Closing the door.

I don't want to be hurt again.

I must shut them out.

Shut them out completely.

I have learnt to loathe.

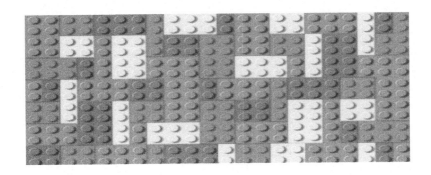

James doesn't say much, but he is sensitive, and knows what's going on.

At the get go, James told Derek and I that what Summer had, was the same thing he had. James at this time was suffering from anxiety. Unfortunately, a change of schools didn't work out, even though the move was carefully considered and we believed it was the best decision - it just didn't work out that way. My very sensitive 9 year old son was now being diagnosed with anxiety /depression/ADD/ and his tests showed high functioning Aspergers, now known as broad spectrum autism. My baby son was categorised as high risk of suicide. He was struggling with being on this planet, at the same time Summer came home with Anorexia.

Okay, back to what James continued to say -
The 2 "A's" are the same Mum.
Right - tell me then son!
And this is what he told me.

The worry of food for Summer is like the worry for me, going to school.

The worry of being fat for Summer, is like the worry for me with new situations.

The worry of calories and eating non-fat anything for Summer, is like the worry for me being in the spotlight.
James, like Mia watched on as our family went into crisis mode and although they were constantly guided by us and the therapy team in family counselling sessions, it was a very difficult and emotionally draining time. James remained quiet most of the time in family counselling sessions, and unfortunately the one time he had something to add to the conversation, he was brushed over by the therapist and as a

result he refused to participate ever again. He refused to come into the room and remained out in the waiting room. After a while, both Mia and James refused to attend the weekly family counselling sessions so Mia looked after James at home while Derek and I took Summer to the hospital.

It took a whole year for James' to feel settled and secure again. It was just awful for him and us too for that matter. There were times the struggle was more difficult with James than the horrific days we were having with Summer. James remains angry with Summer and blames Summer for destroying (his words) our family.

James misses his sister. Summer and James were good mates who played and played and played. They were very close and as a result of the Anorexia, James genuinely suffered from grief due to the loss of his sister. This bond is going to take some time to restore.

I have explained as best as I can to Summer, she is very patient but there are days she is unable to fathom what 'Anna' has done not only to her but to the rest of the family.

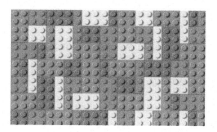

No Space for Words

The dead silence in the car

driving home after family therapy.

The constant battle and compromise over recovery.

The undecided path that is yet to be chosen.

Numbers control my life now.

I live by numbers.

Talking about my feelings

Isn't going to help speed up recovery.

All I need is time.

And time, is all it will take.

They are trying to take control

Away from Anna, from me.

I want them to help,

But this isn't the way.

If they want to help me,
They need to listen to me.

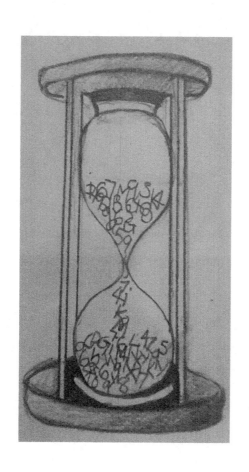

Diary extract by Grace

July 31ˢᵗ

A Letter You Never Want To Find

I found a note on my pillow tonight from Summer. Not the normal ones that I used to get with pretty drawings of flowers with both of us wearing yellow dresses with big smiles on our faces.

No, tonight I received a suicide note saying how much she loved us and that it's just too hard, with a resounding Goodbye.

Needless to say, from here on in, Summer slept on a mattress in our bedroom. It probably marks the time when I stopped sleeping.

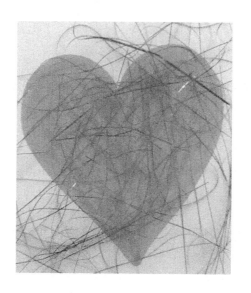

Food Fight

I'm currently sitting at my dining table supervising my daughter to ensure she doesn't make a run for it.

You see, yesterday at the hospital family therapy session I was instructed to feed Summer more food, as in double what I would normally feed her, as she needed to put on more weight.

It is now after lunch and I'm being told how I'm killing her because I want her to eat yogurt. It's been 1.5 hours now, she is very angry with me, I have been yelled at, put down, told how much I don't care about her, how she hates being at home, how it isn't fair. She is crying uncontrollably, she's refusing to do what I ask now, and now saying why can't I just get rid of her. This is such an illogical argument - now I can't back down from my first instruction because as soon as I do she will gain control over her food intake and anorexia will win again.

Don't get me wrong, I'm all for compromise, but we aren't dealing with the "norm" - this is a definite battle of wills between parent and child re-establishing the hierarchy, a parent taking responsibility for their child and I can assure you if you ever considered yourself your daughter's best friend as some Mothers do - the friendship will be broken. You cannot take on the authoritative role and be a friend at the same time. You need to step up and save your child.

Heart break can only describe my emotional state.

I will not give up on my daughter.

Dad's Take

Grace and I run a business from home, which helped enormously, as I could be available to assist Grace with supervising Summer when she had to do all of the other every day running around for home, her work, extended ageing family and everything else concerning James and Mia. Unfortunately, for us, it seemed that all the hospital appointments that suited our timetable were never available. Anyway, Summer on numerous occasions would come out to my converted garage that is now the office, telling me how bad and mean Mum was.

I fell into the trap.

I got sucked into the vortex of Anna, I wanted to play good cop. Not only was Anna winning the battle but Grace and I were at odds. I was trying to be Mr Fix it. Stay in good with Summer and beat Anorexia.

We would go through diets, exercise programs you name it. At the end of the day Summer's brain was more like mashed potato. Nothing was ever retained. Anna was ever present and always listening.

Good cop... Ha... Summer was manipulating me to take sides, and I did. As you can imagine the outcome for me or the family unity wasn't a good one.

Diary extract by Grace

August 3rd

Tired

Last night I just needed to be still and quiet - my head was buzzing, my ears were ringing, I was sick and tired of talking.

You must do

What you think

You cannot do.

- Eleanor Roosevelt-

Introducing Anna

In an attempt to try something different, Summer and I decided to call anorexia Anna ... Give it a name and a face then declare it as the enemy.

I really wanted to reiterate to her that we, as in her parents, family, doctors, counsellors, psychiatrists, nurses, the hospital and moreover food were not the enemy but rather that Anna, so entrenched in her mind was making all the decisions and planning all the fights on behalf of Summer.

The Counselling team at the hospital kept saying - refuse to argue with anorexia, it's the condition that's talking, not Summer.

Easier said than done!

Summer and I went into our back yard and told "Anna" that she was not welcome in our home, that she could no longer come to play and we told her sternly to leave right now.

It felt good to do this at the time. If you are wondering what happened next - "Anna" was listening and WWIII was declared the next morning.

That Scene Does Not Belong To Us

One time I was visiting Summer in hospital and there was a meeting in a room across the hall - parents, doctors, counsellors and the young anorexic patient.

All of a sudden there was screaming, a door slamming and loudly yelled colourful words with the statement "I hate you". A young 15 year old came stomping back to the ward where Summer and I were sitting quietly. I remember feeling sorry for the parents and thinking that surely wouldn't happen to us.

I'm here to tell you, it happened today. I'm numb, I'm speechless, I feel like I've been slapped senseless then left to bleed.

It's time for my daily mantra

I will not give up on my daughter.

A
Summer
Storm

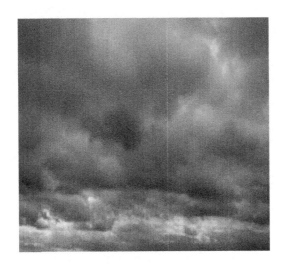

Clouds

The unfairness of no choice

The panic of order

And the absence of normality.

Being normal is the most abnormal behaviour of

the 21st century!

For a while, I wouldn't mind being boring

I miss the ongoing routine of school

The constant laughter of friends.

I can't wait 'til life, freedom, teenage hood

becomes

a part of my vocabulary once again.

My eyes haven't seen the real world for weeks

My heart hasn't felt whole in months

And my life will stay like this for years

I need a miracle

I need someone to save me from this life.

I'm sick of living
I need to help myself
I need to do this alone
I want to do this alone

But the dramatic changes of thought
Is what I beckon for,
It's not what I deserve.

I owe my life and soul to my beautiful family.

But they need to know that this is a journey that I must
travel,
This is my road to self- discovery.

But what does discovery mean?

I don't know.

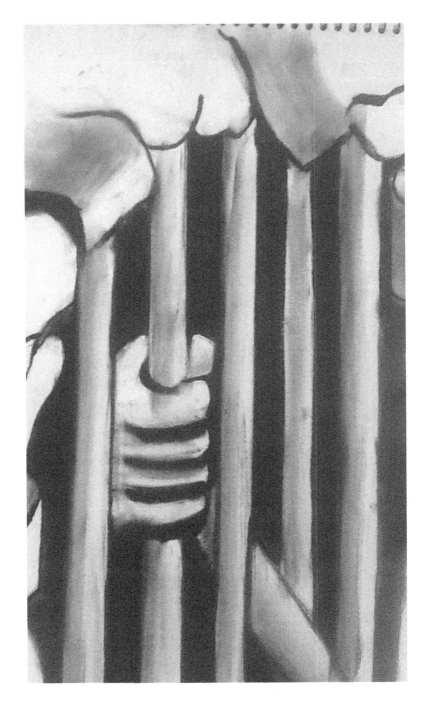

140

Struggles of an Outpatient

We are currently at the hospital, 3 days out of 7, even though we, or I should say Summer, is classified as an outpatient.

Our last visit and weigh in had Summer posting a 250gm loss - how that happened I will never know, so now we are on notice, which means, everytime we have an appointment, we are to bring an overnight bag, as re-admittance is on the cards.

We are now back to the range of Hospital admission - all that work and heartache for nothing. We have 2 days to get weight on, but her temperature is down and she potentially needs hospital care again.

I have her on 24 hour watch - I don't take my eyes off her. I don't let her choose food or make any decision concerning food. I follow her to the bathroom (she knows I'm outside the door). Summer sleeps in my bed so I can ensure she isn't exercising through the middle of the night - the rules are Derek's and my rules so if we say wear socks and put a jumper on, she must comply.

I really do believe we can beat this - her mental health has improved since being at home... Yes she is sneaky, yes Anna is always hovering trying to find other ways to undermine Summer and us - we aren't just dealing with our unwell little girl anymore.

Like Dorothy said to Toto - "I don't think we are in Kansas anymore!"

Tomorrow the family is off to the hospital for our weekly family therapy session. I haven't spoken much or at all how "Anna" has impacted the rest of the family - I will a little later ... But right now I'm uncertain if my little baby princess will be returning home tomorrow or will be re-admitted to hospital.

I am absolutely out of my depth, the counsellor told me to be prepared to have my heart broken, I can assure you it has happened and there will be many more times my heart is smashed relentlessly against the jagged rocks of life before this journey is over.

Mia Talks About

Family Therapy

As much as I would have just loved to move away - and sometimes I was very, very, very close, I would always just hover, just in case.

So I stayed, because deep inside (deep, deep inside) I felt that this anorexia was my fault and it was my responsibility to get rid of it, since I'm the older one and I'm meant to look after everyone younger than me.

Don't ask me why I felt that way! Though it didn't take me long to figure out that thinking that way was absolutely ridiculous and in some ways mental.

That's right. I was living with an anorexic sister and a borderline autistic brother and I was feeling like the mental one! Yep! That sounds about right.

I think for me, the worst part of this whole experience was when the therapy began. I'm not saying therapy was bad or anything like that! It helped a lot in some cases and it absolutely put some uncertainty to rest.

But it was around the time after Summer came home from hospital when the idea of killing her in her sleep came into play.

Dad's Take

If you think you have ever been put under a microscope, just wait for family therapy.

I remember a time in one of our earlier sessions where we had to bring lunch in and eat it in front of the psych team. All was fne until they dissected what had just been consumed. "Do you think that was sufficient?" they asked. All of a sudden you start questioning yourself. "Well obviously not" by the tone of their question. They then asked us what we would like to see Summer eat as a treat. We had to then go to the cafeteria and purchase a treat each. Grace bought her a strawberry milk whilst I chose a chocolate Freddo frog. Summer drank the milk reluctantly but when I produced the chocolate, all hell broke loose.

The tears, the anger, I had never seen anything like it.

Summer had to take a bite. There was no backing down. She bit off a piece 1/3rd of the size of your little finger nail, it was like battery acid on her tongue. Something, only 2 months previous she would have fought you over.

We learnt a lot that day.

In fact, through family therapy we learn a lot every day.

Fight

If I was to be asked

today

to define

anorexia nervosa

in

five

words

I would say

Possessive

Controlling

Strong

Relentless

Unforgiving

There are probably many other words but it's not fixing the problem is it? It's just me venting. It is unbelievably hard to watch my little girl being overrun by an entity nobody invited and one that my husband and I cannot fight.

This is totally her fight. We are instructed by a team of Psychologists, Doctors and Psychiatrists at the Children's Hospital to not let Summer have her say with what, how much and when she eats - our job is to reduce the guilt and take control away from Anna ...

But when your child refuses to eat what do you do?

The family can sit at the dining table for 2 or more hours encouraging Summer to eat but meanwhile my young 9 year old son and 15 year old daughter need to leave the table and systematically attempt to clean up the kitchen, adopting a significant burden of stress themselves in the hope of normalising the routine before their own bedtime.

Okay, Summer needs to finish her dinner - do we sit on her and shovel the food down her throat? Even though you would love to, as isn't this the problem anyway?

FOOD ! FOOD ! FOOD !

If only the grey matter in her brain was functioning normally, her brain has shrunk to the point that she has become mentally unstable. Anorexia is considered a mental health illness.

Previously I mentioned a ski trip, Summer cannot remember any of it. She cannot remember her first three days in hospital when she was admitted. A whole lot of memory is not there, a whole lot of her life is missing. I have stopped taking photos, I have stopped seeing acquaintances, I have become more solitary and introspective. It's a condition that exists but is unspoken and unacknowledged - it's a shameful thing that occurs - it's why we all withdraw.

Today is my sister's birthday, I didn't forget, important people to me are still a priority. It's just that I am so tired and there's just not much left of me to give out to anyone else anymore.

If Only Wishes Came True

I thought I could cope.
I thought that I could.

I thought that I was moving forward.
Moving forward at a steady pace.
Moving forward towards re-establishing
Something that I used to have.
Something that I long for.

Don't think that I'm turning away
Because I can't do it.
I can't carry on.

I'm turning away because it's too hard.

I can't do this life any longer

The label.

The constant mind game.

The control.

The control I don't have.

The control I want and the control I need.

People think they understand.

People think that it's easy for me to accept

The help of others

But I'm the one

And only one

To blame for this situation.

The one extremely difficult to shake.

I wish that this part of my short life was over,

That this dreaded story that I'm living becomes a

distant memory,

A memory that I forbid to revisit.

One that shall be forever locked away

I need a miracle.

I need to be saved.

I need someone to tell me it's okay.

I need it to be someone that I believe.

Someone that I believe I can trust.

I want everything to be okay,

I want everything to fall into place as before.

Close to perfect.

Instead I waste away days of my life.

The ones to spend with friends.

The ones at school.

Or the ones where you fall asleep

To the sound of your math teacher's drone.

I've been doing nothing for so long now

I have lost that spark

That appetising look at life.

If only wishes came true...

A wish that I knew would never come.

This isn't a decision of life or death,
This is a choice between who I am and who I was...

A decision I avoid.

I don't understand why my thoughts are totally
consumed by food,
The need to deceive others about food.

I know I'm thinking them
I don't know why I'm thinking them
But the frightening thing is,
I can't stop.

I can't seem to contain the thoughts that take over my
mind and the way it works.
The replacement of images in the mirror,

What is and what I see.

A migraine that never ends.

A migraine relective of depression, dimension

and deception

A migraine full of Anna.

A bully

A friend

A housemate

An enemy

A killer

Am I suicidal?

I'm doing it slowly. Painfully.

Hard to understand, hard to explain.

It's just a thought that takes you to somewhere no one

wants to be.

I feel trapped.

Caged in. Closed.

No where to run.
No one to talk to.
No one who doesn't judge.

That is the feeling I have,
Every second of every minute
Every hour of every day.

If you haven't lived through it

Then

DON'T

ever

say

you

understand!

I'm done

Done for

Done

Dead

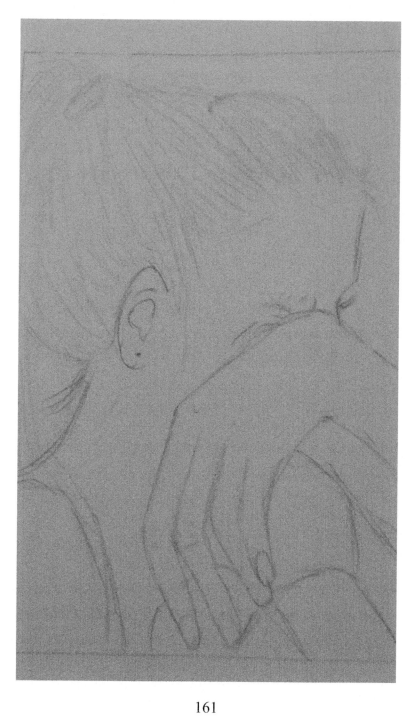

161

Mia Reflects on a

Hellish Day!

Holy Mother!

How do I even explain this?

It was torture.

You feel like you are in a movie – the cliché and cheesy film where everything seems like it's dragging you to hell, but all of a sudden, a hot guy from a foreign country comes and rescues you, and you live happily ever after!

Except for me, it's just the first part - the hot accent guy hasn't popped his head in and said hello yet. Okay, so everything is going to hell and it just keeps going. There's fighting, screaming and peas and chips are thrown all over the place.

Normally, as much as I would have loved to join in on the food fight, I stayed in my place and listened to Jason Mraz and Ed Sheeran sing to their little hearts content, like a loner in my room.

Insight

One of the bizarre thoughts that occur to Anorexia sufferers is that even the smell and fumes of food cooking has calories. We have only learnt about this little treasure recently, and how the same thought carries through to water.

So if you notice your child escaping from the kitchen when preparing the evening meal, chances are, they think they are breathing in weight.

A Shocking Comparison

I was trying to explain the grief we are experiencing to a friend recently and considered very briefly that perhaps if Summer had cancer - it would be easier to deal with.

We could all fight the battle together. We would be on the same side. With anorexia, it is Summer's battle and she keeps Derek and I away, as we are the enemy trying to keep her alive.

Come What May

Every morning I wake up and wonder what the day will bring and how much yelling and upset I will need to endure from my daughter today.

Some days are easier than others.

There is a saying I heard recently -

You are only as happy

as your

unhappiest child.

A card I received in the mail today from
my Sister Marnie

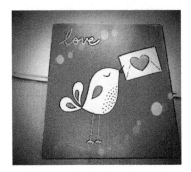

Dear Grace and Derek,

You two have been in my thoughts a lot the past few months as you keep moving your family forward to a better place.

The journey we take as parents never ends the way we planned it out, and how can it when our children take on their own direction and thoughts (and mistakes).

We are catalysts at times it seems. In saying that, you seem to have had more than your fair share to manage, but remember you are not alone. Derek, you are so right when you say it takes a village to raise a child – always know you are both loved and appreciated by all of your family, not just your kids. You are wonderful parents and you know the best way to handle things despite all the well intentioned advice I'm sure you get.

Don't doubt yourselves and don't allow yourselves to feel you didn't get it right.

It's not about you – it's about the journey your lovely children have taken you on, as mine do for me. None of us are out of the woods yet with the next generation but we just need to remember, even on the hardest days, to love them, love each other and support each other, keep guiding them and hope 10% of what we teach our children makes some difference.

Sending you lots of my love today,

Marnie xx

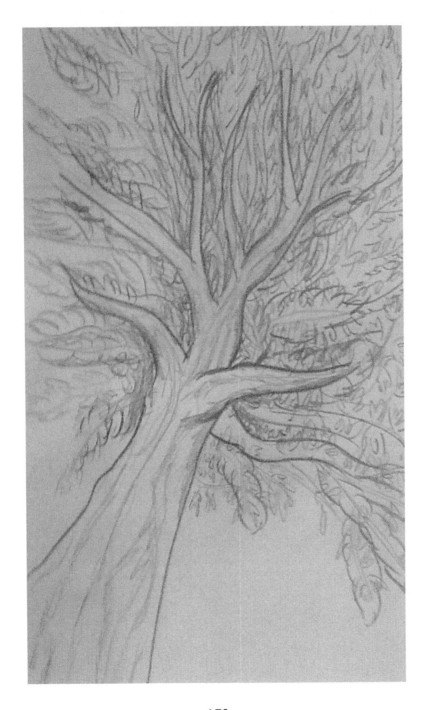

172

Tree

I was explaining to my sister the other night how I'm so tired and spent and used the analogy that I feel like a tree stripped of its bark, however, still standing, but raw with emotion and extremely vulnerable.

In regards to the bark, it's like the bark has been my badge of honour, skills learnt, confidence, achievements and the things I have, most importantly my children, husband, family and friendships. Here on one hand I have friends dubbing me "Mother of the Year" whilst on the other hand my own confidence in mothering and as a person has been rocked so much that at times I'll hesitate in making the easiest of decisions. As a woman and a mother, I always felt I knew what I was doing - always confident to find a solution, always prepared to learn and find better ways of doing things - well my bark is gone and I need to rebuild myself.

After all the research, reading and living with anorexia, I still wonder and have concerns what is my part in all of this. Some 'experts' put it down to poor communication and problem solving skills within the family. Other experts say that anorexia stems from the need to maintain control and the sufferer has low esteem. I'm so frustrated hearing that my child has mental health issues. Everything I thought I knew - I don't - I really am learning to walk again.

As for my sister, she was concerned for me, but I reminded her that I'm not running away (as trees can't) and that even though I have no bark it doesn't mean I will fall over.

I'm not sure of my point

other than

you can't give up

even if you want to.

Another Day

My mother got burnt

Burnt by a fire that used to exist
A fire that ran out over time
A fire that is now just a memory
And not a reality
It is a fire that created a scar
A scar of hate.

My Mother is scared
And that scar reminds her of the past.
The scar that needs time to heal
But when she lights the flame and starts a fire
The scar will never have time to heal.

To heal for good.

She not only burns herself

But everyone else around her

A selfish action.

A hurtful action

An action that can cause damage and silence.

Think before you do.

I decided to ignore the injured

To work with the recovered.

When she's away, it is gone

All the stress

All the tears

My concerns disappear

Disappear into thin air.

I can't understand

Her motive to destroy my journey of recovery

She is unscrewing the train track

Letting the rails loose.

She has a new form of the disease

It's not eating

It's destroying.

Destroying the stairs I built.

The stairs I'm no longer able to climb

But I am running, running as fast as I possibly can.

Why is she making it so hard?

I am scarred from the damage that has occurred.

Yet I know it will take longer for Mum

to heal than me.

Days are finally starting to get back to normal.

And those days

are

the days

with Dad.

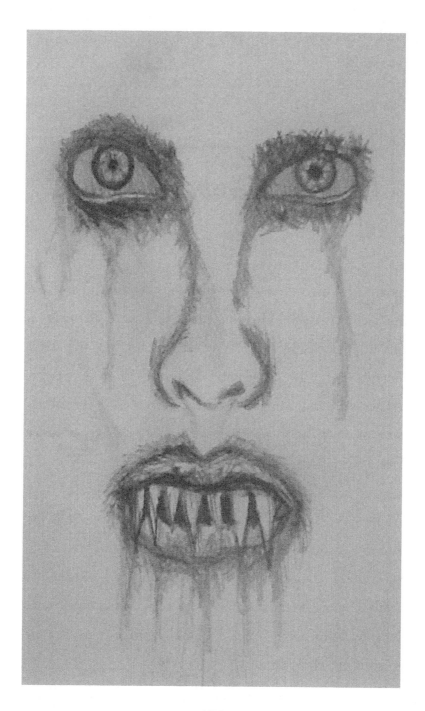

It's a Numbers Game

By all accounts we would now be considered in phase 2 of the recovery stage. The emergency is over - Summer is currently medically stable. We are part of the outpatient program of the hospital. Summer's heart, weight, temperature and urine is tested every week - sometimes twice a week and we meet with the psych team every Monday.

We have decided not to let Summer know her weight as she is clearly distressed with any gain and the ensuing week is a full throttle anorexia melt down- with tears, screaming, reduced eating, exercise, refusing to keep warm, depression, defiance, being more secretive and all in all a pretty crappy time for the whole family.

Summer is focused on numbers and time.

Summer clock watches until her next meal, it has to be served at the exact time every day or she becomes agitated and paces around the house like a caged lion.

Any packets, cartons, bottles and boxes are scrutinised for their nutritional value, fat content and calorie count.

Summer has been banned from the pantry, to prevent her from fervently studying all of the labels.

Summer cannot go into a supermarket. The last time I took her she raced around reading all the labels and constantly disappeared to touch, look and smell the food she so needs, but won't have. It was alarming and sad to watch her; she was crazed and frenzied surrounded by all this food.

Meal times continue to be stressful, she watches me from the corner of her eye analysing how much and what I am preparing. Summer is constantly ready to pounce if she feels I am trying to manipulate her food intake.

Our life is focused on Summer's weight.
If it is up, down or the same.

If it is down, we have failed.

If it is up, we fail

in our daughter's eyes as

she believes we are

hurting her.

1234567891011213

14151617181920212

22324252627282930

29282726252423222

12019181716151413

12111098765432101

23456789987456321

1234567891011213

14151617181920212

This is an email received from Derek's Sister

Dear Grace and Derek,

I wanted to write and let you know how I feel about Summer's progress. When you both say, it's Summer who has been the achiever in all of this, you are right but not completely.

When I was heart broken, no one could have fixed that except me. That said, my journey was made so much easier with the support of my family and friends. I don't believe I would be feeling as emotionally well as I do, without that support. You let me talk, cry a little and little by little I mended.

The same in my mind is unequivocal of Summer. With you both, with the support you have enlisted, with the lengths you have gone to, she seems to be turning a huge corner and starting to mend as well.

If my family and friends had made light of feelings and been glib and unsupportive, no doubt I would have gotten there but in much less style and grace. It's been your unrelenting commitment to Summer, your can do attitude and untiring efforts, that have taken Summer from where she started this dark chapter five months ago, to where she is now.

The combination of all this and no doubt much more has turned your beautiful princess around. I am sure you are still on tenterhooks, thinking any day Anna will return and rightfully so. But from what I could more than casually observe, you, your family and precious Summer has beaten the best of this and Anna is now simply withering whilst Summer now prospers.

My congratulations aren't necessary and would be trite but not my admiration of the both of you. You are stunning parents and the love that exudes from your children towards you both, is testimony of that. They want to be near you and interact with you. I found myself on more than one occasion, being halted by such overt affection and respect given by them.

Grace and Derek, these are not just words, this is what I've seen repeatedly and I have no doubt about my summation.

Vigilance, closeness and consistency are just three of the myriad requisites to raising a family successfully and whilst there are plenty of trying times in between that give cause for doubt, just look at what you are doing and have done thus far and stand tall and be proud of yourselves. As I said earlier, you are stunning parents and if there is a book in either of you, then let it be a "how to" of successful parenting.

You have earned my unbridled respect and you two are the most deserving parents going.

To both of you, simply but fully, bravo.

Tess

Diary extract by Grace

November 3rd

Family

Whilst all the books advise to keep a united front, stay firm and not give in to the demands, it is not always easy when there are four other people living in the house. As parents protecting and guiding Summer through this we know we have compromised our other 2 children and they are hurting.

They cannot understand and our eldest daughter has become angry with Summer for what she is doing to herself, for what she is doing to our family, the selfishness of anorexia and the stupidity of it all.

Mia is afraid of being Summer's big sister and being responsible for her. Mia is adamant that she doesn't want Summer to go to her school again.

Yesterday, I suggested the girls go for a wander for an hour at a large shopping mall close by home, Mia was afraid to be with Summer on her own, in case there was a meltdown. After lots of talking and trying to console both girls, they went for an hour and had a nice time.

Both girls clearly had missed their relationship, the camaraderie and the same interests in music, shows and drawing. It was important for them as much as me and for our family that the girls restored some sense of sisterhood. It is not easy but through all of this, they are stronger and more understanding of each other's challenge with Anna.

James is hurting too. He is a sensitive little boy who feels the heaviness in the air, sees the tear in my eye and hears the constant sharp tongue of his sister berating me for insisting she eats something. I am so sorry how hurtful this is to Mia and James. I am trying to do more for them, but it isn't enough. I am giving them more attention and time, but it isn't enough. I'm cuddling them more, but it isn't enough.

After Summer's attempt to run away, James hasn't slept well, he is frightened she will jump out of the window and disappear through the night. He is refusing to go to school because he feels he needs to watch her. His anxiety is at extreme levels. It is a mess.

We are a family in crisis.

I told Mia and James that their job was to play and be on their sisters side and that it was Derek's and my responsibility to look after, watch and keep Summer safe.

This helped a bit.

We also let them decide if they wanted to attend the hospital therapy sessions, allowing them to have a much needed break. It was against the Maudsley approach, and we continually apologised to Annaleise for their absence but we had three unhappy children. If I could repair two immediately, then that was what I was going to do.

Now it is rare that the five of us go into the hospital together. Generally, Derek and I take turns which means one of us is at home to help with homework and organise dinner.

Summer understands and knows that she has her siblings love and support. She recognises that when they don't come to the hospital it is because they must lead their own lives. Ironically, this has allowed Summer to take responsibility of "Anna" and push harder to re-join the family.

I think Summer is sorry for the pain she causes her brother and sister on a daily basis. Yet she is not truly aware of her thoughts and actions and thus I believe an apology is not necessary from her.

Maybe when this is all over, Summer may feel the need to apologise to her siblings privately.

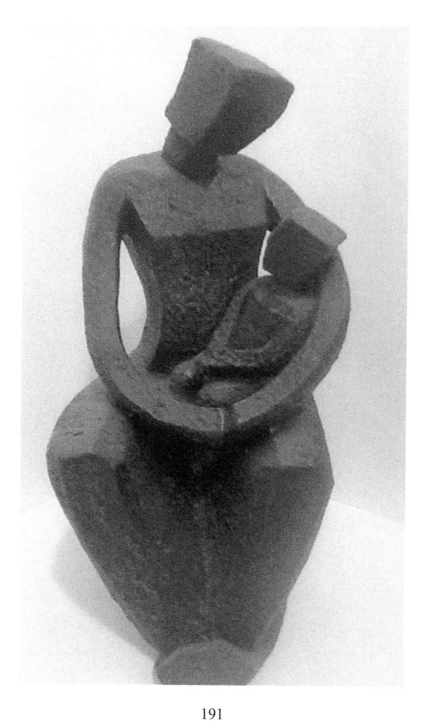

It Just Has To Be Said!

It pains me to write this, but I feel I need to for those who have a preconceived idea that Anorexia Nervosa only occurs in attention seeking teenage upstarts.

Anorexia is a medical condition, a taboo subject that is often unacknowledged. It is perceived by many as a shameful 'thing' that leads people to gossip as if your child was a drug addict, or a thief or a murderer.

Some of Derek's and my family members are angry with Summer as they feel she has full control and knowledge of what she is doing to this family. They believe Summer can turn this 'thing' off! Many times we have heard how she is a selfish, manipulative spoilt brat. What do we do with people like that? You keep your child away from them, that's what. Summer does not need negativity and neither do we.

I have found myself and still do, making up some story as to why Summer is not at school, is in hospital or not looking very well. You can't stop people talking, but the rumour mongers, both children and adults around the school grounds are sometimes too much to bear. I don't need this grief, nor does my family; I am much too tired to take people to task about their ignorance.

I would like to set the record straight and straighten out all of the misconceptions of Anorexia Nervosa right now!

Anorexia Nervosa is not something you ask for

People with anorexia do eat

Anorexia is curable

Anorexic sufferers are not all thin and emaciated

Anorexia is a condition that describes the refusal to eat, however, it is the reasons for the refusal or restrictive intake of food that is the underlying problem.

Emotional dysfunction can lead to the misuse of food.

For the comfort eaters out there I hope you can relate to this description. You know the ones who will tuck into a tub of ice-cream or load up on chocolate because they are feeling a bit down? Oprah Winfrey is a fully confessed comfort eater. Well, there are always two sides, the Yin and the Yang - is one better than the other?

There are three distinct aspects of diagnosing Anorexia Nervosa.

The **physical** aspect may include weight loss, amenorrhea (the loss or abnormal absence of menstruation) fainting and cold intolerance.

The **behavioural** aspect may include strict dieting, secretive eating, binge eating, compulsive exercise, laxatives, diet pills or diuretic abuse, impaired relationships, withdrawing socially and signs of Obsessive Compulsive Disorder.

The **emotional** aspect may include depression, anxiety, low self esteem, fear of weight gain and body image distortion.

So back to the knockers and the hecklers who are too scared to jump into our arena. My baby nearly died. Her heart was failing. She is sick.
She is experiencing one of the loneliest journeys you could ever take.
Summer is not the same person.

I am sad, I miss her. I know I am suffering with grief. Every relationship in my home is stressed and suffering. I will not give up on my daughter.

So for those of you who asked what did I do to cause this? Suggested that this illness is my or Derek's fault, or said to leave her to suffer the consequences, or blamed Summer, or stayed away because it got too hard.

This statement is for you –

If you can't
stand by US
at OUR low points
then don't think
you can enjoy
OUR successes.

Much of the Same

Life has settled down a bit now. Summer is trying very hard, every minute of the day. She eats what is given to her without complaint and she is attempting to read, draw and is co-writing this book.

Summer has always maintained that only she can fix this problem. Not us, not the Doctors or Psychologists. She is the one who decides when to eat, Summer is adamant that we have had nothing to do with her recovery, nor can we take credit for her weight gain.

This is correct in part, however, for anyone to get through Anorexia, they do need love, care, unconditional support and kindness. What I say now may seem patronising but ultimately when your child is screaming at you, you as the parent just have to let it wash over. Do not fight with Anorexia, it is psychotic and you will lose. Believe me, this is not easy and causes emotional damage.

Routines have been re-established at home, but we are still taking Summer to the hospital once or twice per week. Calm has been restored and Mia and James are less shell shocked. Mia has started to invite her friends home again which tells me she is feeling more settled with home life.

Constant positive communication and checking in with Mia and James has helped. Fielding their often raw questions was necessary.

For Summer the constant conversation of food, weight, meal plans and "Anna" was not helping. We decided as a family, to stop talking about 'it'. This strategy helped. Our work load is still similar to that of when we were in crisis mode, however, I think we are just coping better, we have accepted our lot in life and don't complain. Our heads are clearer and even though I am up at 3am writing this story whilst everyone else is fast asleep, I find it therapeutic and there are less restless nights for my family.

There are always different ways to skin a cat - sorry for all of you cat lovers, we do have a cat! What I mean is, if you are fortunate to have been accepted into the "system", like we were, unfortunately it means your child was very sick, so sick that they were accepted into a 12 bed maximum hospital ward facility. That's right; we only have 12 beds available for eating disorder patients at Westmead Children's Hospital!

On clinic days at the Hospital, when you see all the families and their kids with Anorexia turn up to get weighed and counselled, you realise we have an epidemic. What is sadder is that it is the same families' week in, week out. It doesn't take long to realise that you are on this treadmill wondering if your daughter will ever get better. It reminds me of that movie with Jack Nicholson who suffered from OCD, his remark to a room full of patients waiting to see a therapist, was "what if,

   this is

    as good

     as it gets?"

I am now recalling one of our first hospital family therapy sessions where I was asked how I would feel if we were in the same place a year from now. I almost fell off my chair and was unable to process that comment for a couple of days. Unfortunately, it is a valid question.

Another method treating Anorexia is to send the patient away for therapy and re-feeding programme for a 6 week to 3 month period. The "better" places can range anywhere from $1,000 AUD to a whopping $5,000 AUD per day!

It is the mindset behind these other forms of therapy that bother me most as the premise seems to be that parents are the instigator, or partly responsible for the reason their child has developed Anorexia. So in other words, their mission is to remove the child from home to save them, from you. In some cases, it might have some truth, but mostly I find this archaic and unfair. These programmes unwittingly perpetuate the myth that it is the parents or families fault.

There is nothing wrong with other styles of therapies. In fact I have tried most and am very happy to give feedback via the email site we have set up. Every recovery model is different, so I don't wish to direct or influence the approach you are taking in helping your child recover.

When life presents challenges - it is not necessarily how you deal with them, but rather what you learn about yourself along the way.

It is being prepared to face the problem, rather than hide from them that ultimately make the difference.

Summer's Account

Games That Are Frowned Upon

I cheated the system.

I'm cheating myself.

It's something that wasn't new

To me or to Anna.

She's lying. I'm lying.

She's not real.

But I am.

I can't bring myself

To the decision of truth.

Calamity will follow

My regretful actions.

I regret making them.

Not doing them.

Unfortunate.

But not tragic.

What's done is done.

The past is unchangeable.

Water is a heavy dense particle.

I was fooled by my unwise demon.

Pressure can be applied anywhere

And everywhere on anything.

I used those two dangerous things

To her advantage.

To my disadvantage.

Those two things I cannot take back.

She makes the decisions,

But I take the fall.

Drink she said, drink.

Pressure she said, pressure.

I hooked my feet under the bar,

The bar of the chair,

The chair that decided
A good week from a bad week.
A chair that told the world my weight.

For three weeks I made a mistake
Pressure and water

Water

Weight

Eventually I was caught,
Caught up in lies
In numbers

In Words

The time had come
I was no longer allowed
To put pressure on the bar
Using my feet.

My lie revealed

I had dropped weight.

A lot of weight!

I Confessed

I couldn't handle

The look of

Disappointment upon their faces.

Distress

A Small Light Appears At The End Of Our Long Dark Tunnel

Now that the heat is off this particular event, I can write about it and share with you what I absolutely believe was the turning point of Summer's road to recovery and kicking Anna to the kerb.

A definite part of anorexia is deceitfulness. Your precious child, who never lied before, will now lie in order for anorexia to win. It is quite disarming because part of you still wants to believe you are being told the truth whilst the other part of you is wary, suspicious and constantly on guard. You, as a parent, just want it all to go away so that you can resume your normal life.

For months we have been visiting the hospital twice a week. Monday's for family therapy with a weigh in, followed by a good hour of talking with our psychologist and then again on Thursday for a weigh in, medical check and a quick consult about life at home for Summer.

For weeks Summer's weight was like a yo yo - up 2kg, down by 2.5kg, down 1.3kg, up 300 grammes yet by all accounts we were following the set instructions. We were preparing food, monitoring her eating, not allowing exercise, no school, making her sleep on a pull out bed in our bedroom and listening for bouts of bulimia at the bathroom door. She was on 24 hour watch.

Derek and I constantly came away from our Monday's meeting at the hospital confused, troubled and alarmed. We were feeling defeated, responsible and ashamed that we could not maintain Summer's weight. What were we doing wrong? Trying to explain ourselves to the Counsellors and Doctors what we were feeding Summer was degrading and deflating. Gone was our once confident approach to parenting.

After some soul searching, I chatted with Derek. We realised we needed a new outlook, not one based on doubting ourselves but one based on encouragement and reinforcement. We needed a plan and we needed it now.

To us the Maudsley approach was fundamentally the best option as we were opposed to sending Summer to another facility away from home and her support network. However, I must stress, that you as the parent/s definitely know your child and do know what's best. Yes, the Doctors are there, but your hourly, weekly appointment is only just that, you are still responsible for the rest of the 7 days / 24 hours.

Finally, we found out why Summer's weight had been so erratic. Apparently, at the time of weigh in, Summer would hook her feet under a bar on the weighing chair and push down to increase her weight. Summer finally admitted to water loading to help tip the scale.

Not forgetting that
1 litre of water = 1 kg of weight.

With that all in the open, I thanked my daughter for being honest and recognised that in revealing her tricks, it meant she wanted us to help her stop these games. Well perhaps!

Partly, it was a definite indication that Summer was fed up with the standing appointment at the hospital, fed up being watched, monitored and psycho analysed 24/7. She had, had enough of having no life and being constantly at home. Summer had been away from school and her friends for 16 weeks.

Other significant factors in helping Summer defeat "Anna" were getting Summer back to school, encouraging her to re-contact and begin networking with friends, allowing her to be social and use her brain. It was definitely hard for Summer, she was very self-conscious and fearful of how her fellow students would judge her. She imagined they would ostracise and reject her. My only advice was "to fake it 'til you make it" - meaning if she acted like she didn't have anorexia, then all those around her would soon forget and stop watching her. This is exactly what they did.

A major obstacle was lunch time. I was absolutely prepared to drive to school and sit in the car with her while she ate her lunch. Summer pleaded that this not happen, as she was concerned this would result in the other students laughing or mocking her. In the end I compromised and gave her a two day trial. There was no weight loss. A correct and untampered weigh in was to be in our favour. Summer kept the privilege and the next four weigh ins showed a weight gain.

At this time, we asked for anti-depressant medication for Summer. This medication takes up to 6 weeks to work effectively - but the results were positive. Her argumentative assaults were reduced and she was beginning to laugh and smile. Summer's conversations and reasoning were more in line to the original Summer. My girl began to play again and most importantly interact with her brother and sister. Our reports to the hospital were more positive than negative. We were reporting minimal arguments with Summer and minimal resistance to eating food. Things were fnally looking up.

Two weeks ago in our counselling session, I commented to our Psychologist that Summer had her appetite back. She was hungry when she came home from school. One of the many things Anorexia does is suppress the automatic response of hunger and appetite.

Summer was beginning to enjoy food, to eat the occasional chip, taste the new type of chocolate that had been bought, and not to fuss or refuse to eat a tub of yogurt or drink cold milk with Milo. Summer, I don't think was bingeing (yet) but the irony of it all, was that I was now starting to say no more food because you will spoil your dinner. How crazy is that?

So here we are in mid-November – exactly four months and two days since Summer was admitted to hospital, now it would seem according to our Psychologist that Summer no longer has Anorexia.
She had beaten and kicked "Anna" to the kerb. I know I cannot get too excited just yet, this ugly and deadly intruder attacked once and I'm concerned if I take my eye off the ball it will attack again.

Summer has defied the odds, books and statistics. Seven years is the average lifespan of this disease including more than a year in therapy and ongoing medical checks. For many it remains a part of life. My hope is that Summer has defeated the spell – that my child is truly strong and most extraordinary.

For me , I cannot wait for New Year's Eve to click over to the next year, so I can say good riddance to this shocking year my Summer, my family and myself have experienced.

But please, no matter how awful it gets,
do not give up on your daughter.

Advice From a Use To Be

If you suffer from this disease,

I know how much pain you are experiencing.

I know how many tears you have shed.

You will get through this.

You are strong.

You are your own person.

Only you control you.

Don't be a coward

Don't back away from a battle

That you might not know you can win.

You will reach the other side.

You will find that better, stronger, healthier person

You once knew.

You will be someone who now values life,
No longer wanting it gone.

Keep Going

You Can

You Will

You Just Need To Try

Trust ME

The Return of Summer

I'm back.

And I'm here to stay.

Stay forever.

It's been a long road.
One that I could not have completed
Without the support
The guidance of my family.
They are my whole world.

I've found my laugh,
I have found my smile.
My little world is no longer crumbling
It is mending

It is a time of renewal.

I didn't ever think my new found thoughts
would be so clear.

I thought my life could never return to normal
Knowing what I've done in the past.

But I did. I did it.

It is possible.

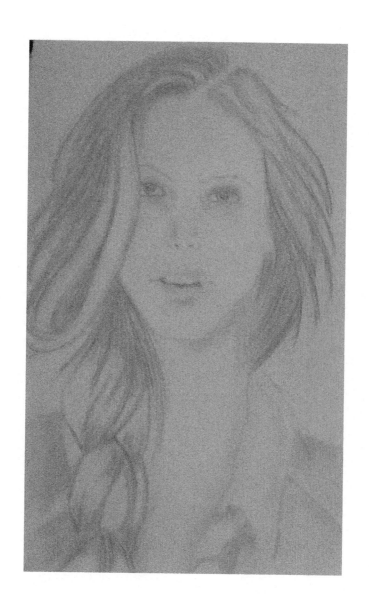

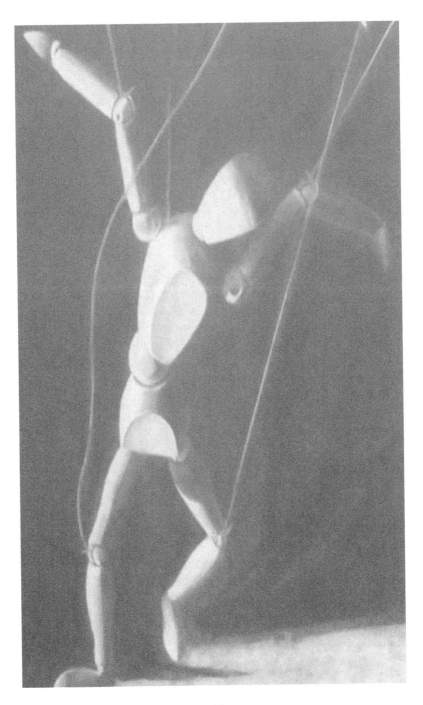

222

Guilt Trip

I've put my family through hell.

I've made them cry.

I've made them smile.

I've made them disappointed.

But I've also made them proud.

I'm sorry.

The rough times.

The good times,

The uneasy times,

The bad times

Throughout this journey.

Thank you, for sticking by me,

I pushed you away from my heart and head.

I let a demon enter our home

Change our family.

When I was yelling,

Screaming,

Fighting

I didn't realise who was talking,

Who was yelling,

Who was screaming,

Who was telling me to fight.

I couldn't separate the two voices.

I have no recollection of my words during these fights.

I have no recollection because they weren't my own

thoughts.

They were hers.

I'm not shifting the blame,

I'm not saying I'm not guilty,

I'm saying that I was controlled.

I was her puppet and she pulled the strings.

People might say it was easy,
But this was the hardest thing
I've ever had to do.

It's more cowardly submitting
To an eating disorder
Than fighting one.

.

.

.

.

I'm not a coward.

.

.

.

.

Believe in Yourself

The dark times are now over,

The sad times have left,

And Anna is gone.

For the last and final time,

I am Summer

Just a normal teenager,

Who has gone through an

Abnormal experience.

No longer two people,

Just one.

I have my personality back

I have found my inner strength.

If I can do it, you can.

You are beautiful, believe it.

Never back, but somewhat here.

I don't know when it will stop.
I don't know if it will.
But let's hope someday it might.

I wasn't easy, it isn't easy.

If only this day was a memory
Instead of a reality.

That has consumbed my life
Seemingly

Forever.

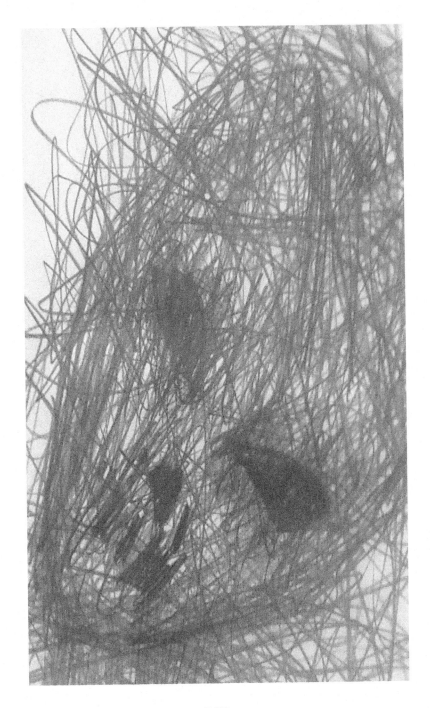

228

Summer's Reality Check

The first half of my story,

I don't remember writing,

Thinking

or

Feeling.

People remind me

I was at the snow, or at Luna park

But I have no memory.

I was there

But my head was not.

Memories forever lost.

Dad's Take

Ultimately you need to trust yourself and believe what you are doing is right, except when you are dealing with anorexia nervosa. Help won't come to you. You need to seek it out and quickly. With all due respect we saw two GP's who were both useless. Don't risk it, go straight to a hospital. Grace is a qualified counsellor but she couldn't get a handle on this 'thing', the average punter has no chance!

Although the days are less stressful as Summer is getting stronger, both in mind and body, we as a family are always on the lookout. Christmas Day was particularly hard for Summer. Our beautiful daughter Mia picked that one up. Lots of food, festivities etc. Mum and Dad certainly missed the ball on that one.

James our fantastic little boy is always on the look out for "Anna" and happy to gun her down if she ever raises her head. We expect this journey to continue for a while to come, if nothing else, it has made us stronger and more resilient as a family unit.

Summer has a few OCD tags and as a result "Anna" has been distanced but I know she still sits quietly in the corner waiting to pounce. Anna knows her days are numbered in this house.

It is through the constant assistance of Jo, Dr Madden, Andrew, Josh, Megan and especially Annaliese that we will one day say goodbye to Anna.

Dad's Take

Trying to keep the wheels on wasn't easy. There were times we just wanted out. The vast majority of our friends and family would call regularly to check on us, which was lovely.

There are sadly a few, to this day who cannot approach the subject of Anorexia with us or Summer. One cannot even bring themselves to read this story.

One of Grace's closet friends said, "what did you do wrong, to cause this." Some family members although sympathetic will judge you, some will live in denial. At the end of the day, all have been ignorant.
The void and isolation of this disease is worrying and all consuming.

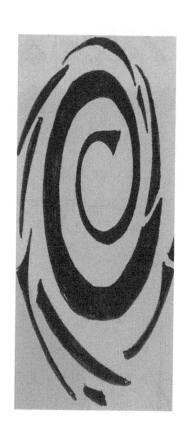

Mia's

Advice on Survival

It's hard to think that I'll ever be at peace with Summer. I'm still angry with her and there have been days where I have gone all day without talking to her.

Like everyone, people have their good and bad days; so far it has been a long string of bad days for me.

If I have any advice or comforting support to anyone who is in a similar situation, have some faith or hope or whatever else there is that keeps you going because even though everything is heading to the crap hole, hopefully your foreign guy or girl will be just around the corner to save you from the depths of hell.

Or even better, stuff the guy, buy yourself a bunch of cats and move out!

I would say good luck, but you are going to need much more than that!

See you on the other side.

Mia x

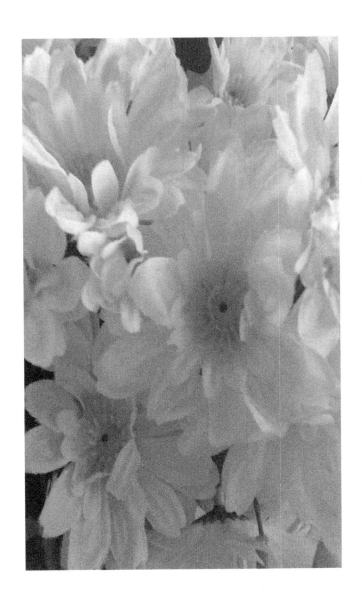

Grace's Reality Check

I know last month I indicated that Summer had turned a corner, the same thoughts echoed in Derek's writings and his actions when he phoned and texted everyone we know saying the nightmare was over and how special and unique Summer was for kicking Anna's butt in record time.

I'm not necessarily a sceptic or known for seeing my glass half empty as opposed to half full. It's just that something isn't quite right and although I keep encouraging Summer, there is something unsettling about her behaviour.

Anna hasn't gone away like everyone seems to think.

We are busily planning for Christmas, all of the family are coming here again. Yes, lunch and beds for 20 guests. Our Christmas celebrations include lunch, dinner, supper then breakfast, lunch and dinner on Boxing Day! I think it would have been a spirited gesture for someone else to take over this year's festivities after the lows of the past months. I'm thinking this, not sure I really mean it!

We have also planned a lovely holiday and intend it to be one that brings the family together and gives us all a chance to really enjoy life.

Last Diary extract by Grace

December 31st

The End

In closing, I just wanted to make you aware that special holidays, family get togethers and parties are ironically a definite trigger for Anna. Christmas in particular! What is there a lot of on Christmas Day apart from presents, good will and crazy Aunties?

Yes, you got it, FOOD, and lots of it.

Summer found it particularly difficult. I did too as I was running around and didn't necessarily have opportunity to watch and check in with Summer as to how much and what she was eating, or more to the point, not eating. She felt that the family would stare at her as they had never seen an anorexic person before. She wasn't far wrong.

I witnessed a friend of Summer's Aunty take a second look, step back while Summer was greeting her Aunty and look from feet to head, I looked on with horror and quickly stepped in the way in the hope of preventing Summer from witnessing this indignity.

The other comments, usually well meaning, but often hurtful come from Aunties, Uncles and Grandparents, as they report how clever they are because they got Summer to eat something. By inference, Derek and I are clearly not clever. The most hurtful comments come when they say throw away lines like, "What is the problem, I don't know why you are complaining how hard it is? Perhaps she should come live with me." My other favourite is, "Stop pestering the poor girl, she will eat when she is hungry."

Stay strong and deflect these unhelpful comments, you know in your heart what is right and what to do. If the answer doesn't come immediately, sleep on it and trust that the appropriate action, answer or solution will present itself in the morning.

Goodnight xx

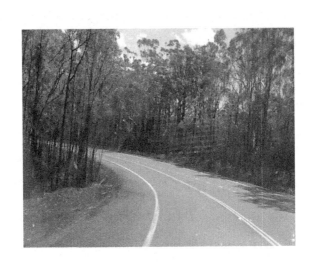

Dad's Take

This is a journey no parent, carer or anyone for that matter should have to take. Eating disorders kill almost as many people per year as smoking related diseases.

But it's never spoken about.

We as parents can be tricky like Anna.

We would be happy to talk to you if you need support or to find out our tricks. Tricks we can't disclose as "Anna" can read too.

annabegone@gmail.com

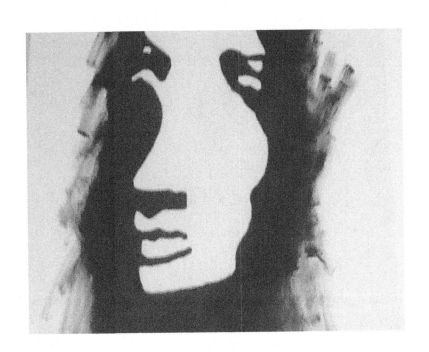

Anna Rexia

R.I.H.

Eulogy written by Grace

H = Hell

Eulogy

Anorexia has gone,

But not forgotten.

You impacted so many lives

Without concern

You have caused untold grief.

You are a powerful entity

You turned up uninvited,

Made a mess, abused our family home.

I will never forgive your attempts to harm my child.

Nothing or no one hurts my child

and gets away with it.

You will never be welcome in our lives,

in our home or in our bodies.

We have turned our back on you,

and have walked away.

You will never find us.

Dad's Final Take

January 1st

The sun on the new year is well and truly up now as I sit and gaze out over the ocean watching the waves roll in.

What a beautiful day it is.
I love my family.

No matter what challenges lay ahead for us, we know that together we can face them.

Together we stand to fight another day.

My glass is now full, looking forward, never back.

Derek

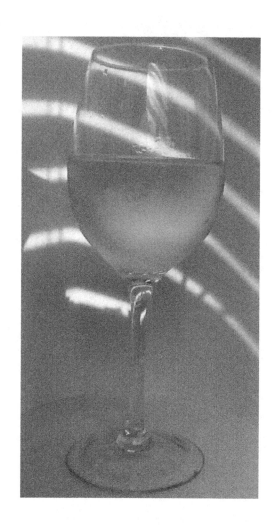

Mia

Has the Last Say

You learn to appreciate good health.

Ultimately, through everything that's happened I have learnt to be grateful for my health and self-control.

It's said that the siblings who live with an anorexic have a 5-10% chance of developing anorexia themselves.

Through his whole affair, that statistic has weighed heavily on my mind and it makes you question yourself.

Am I weak?

In a situation such as this, I have become negative, cynical, hard and almost unemotional.

I haven't allowed myself to cry for 14 months.

You adapt to the heart ache. You learn to say nothing when your parents are discussing her treatment, her eating or just HER. You learn how to show comfort to your Mum when she is sobbing on your shoulder.

Throughout this book, I recorded my inner thoughts and identified my anger towards this whole situation. Towards her.

I am angry that therapy has made me believe that I am at risk to this disease.

I am angry that she is basically a walking corpse.

I am angry that she's ruined every aspect of our family life in this past year.

I'm not afraid to say that now.

Even when I'm writing this, she's screaming at my Mum because she can't have dinner at 6pm.

I blame her for that.

She thinks she doesn't have Anorexia.

I don't believe that Anorexia is a person- when I say her or she - I purely and honestly mean my sister. She got herself into this position and I'm sick of offering my hand and getting it slapped away.

My sister is still sick - and no amount of therapy, meds, empathy or love will make her better.

There comes a time when she has to get off the exercise machine and get out of the house. Preferably to walk down to Coles and buy something that has more than 500KJ.

To the people who think I am weak

You are wrong.

I ignore my life at home because that's how I cope. I give no empathy towards my sister because she has lost all motivation to get better - not because I have given up, she has given up.

I'm afraid that she'll hurt me while I'm asleep yet I manage
to sleep through the night.

I may be angry and I may be lost but

I

Am

Strong

Activities and Discussion Questions for the English Classroom

1. Imagine you are either Mia or James. We gain an understanding of their view points but only in a limited way. How else might their life be affected?

2. How would you respond if you had a brother or sister affected by Anorexia?

3. Summer's contributions are in verse, what might this tell you about the type of person she is?

4. Summer provides no reason as to why she developed the disease and it is clear that other members of the family have been unable to pinpoint the reason. What does this tell you about Anorexia? Has it changed your view on Anorexia?

5. Re-read the entries that deal with the hospital experience. Why is this experience so difficult for every family member?

6. Why does Summer say she is the only one who can fight "Anna"? From reading this book to what extent is this statement true?

7. Research Anorexia and write a factual article about the effects of the disease.

8. Write a letter to Summer expressing your understanding of the situation she faces.

9. Look closely at Summer's drawings, what different moods and inner feelings do they reflect?

10. What is your reaction to reading this true story from each of the family's perspectives?

Index to Summer's Verses

annabegone@gmail.com

has been set up so you can ask questions, share your
story, give feedback on our story or
order a book.

Like the **Annabegone**

page on Facebook

Please follow us on our journey and be
the first to know when Book 2 will be released.

For every copy of this book sold, we are making a
donation to
Westmead Children's Hospital.

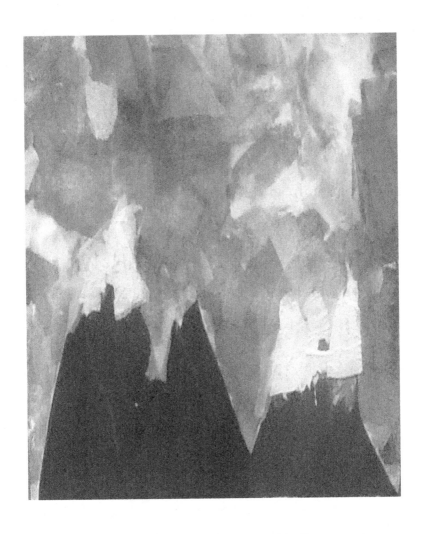

A Cloudy Mountain submitted by James.

Interpretation: Where the beauty of a coloured sky meets the harsh terrain of a black mountain. Even though the peaks are snow capped, I wonder what is more dominating? The light or the dark?

James in art therapy reflected the colour as his family, the snow as the meeting point of where Summer began and the black mountains as Anorexia (Anna) took over – all this from a kid who doesn't like to draw!

Made in the USA
Monee, IL
15 September 2020